# A Review of PAP Therapy for the Treatment of OSA

*Editor*

MATTHEW R. EBBEN

# SLEEP MEDICINE CLINICS

www.sleep.theclinics.com

December 2022 • Volume 17 • Number 4

**ELSEVIER**

1600 John F. Kennedy Boulevard • Suite 1800 • Philadelphia, Pennsylvania, 19103-2899

http://www.theclinics.com

**SLEEP MEDICINE CLINICS Volume 17, Number 4**
**December 2022, ISSN 1556-407X, ISBN-13: 978-0-323-98789-9**

Editor: Joanna Collett
Developmental Editor: Axell Ivan Jade M. Purificacion

*Sleep Medicine Clinics* (ISSN 1556-407X) is published quarterly by Elsevier Inc., 360 Park Avenue South, New York, NY 10010-1710. Months of issue are March, June, September and December. Business and Editorial Offices: 1600 John F. Kennedy Blvd., Ste. 1800, Philadelphia, PA 19103-2899. Customer Service Office: 3251 Riverport Lane, Maryland Heights, MO 63043. Periodicals postage paid at New York, NY and additional mailing offices. Subscription prices are $234.00 per year (US individuals), $100.00 (US and Canadian students), $653.00 (US institutions), $272.00 (Canadian individuals), $267.00 (international individuals), $135.00 (International students), $682.00 (Canadian and International institutions). Foreign air speed delivery is included in all *Clinics* subscription prices. All prices are subject to change without notice. **POSTMASTER:** Send change of address to *Sleep Medicine Clinics*, Elsevier Health Sciences Division, Subscription Customer Service, 3251 Riverport Lane, Maryland Heights, MO 63043. Customer Service: **Tel: 1-800-654-2452 (U.S. and Canada); 314-447-8871 (outside U.S. and Canada). Fax: 314-447-8029. E-mail: journalscustomerservice-usa@elsevier.com (for print support); journalsonline-support-usa@elsevier.com (for online support).**

*Reprints.* For copies of 100 or more of articles in this publication, please contact the Commercial Reprints Department, Elsevier Inc., 360 Park Avenue South, New York, NY 10010-1710. Tel.: 212-633-3874; Fax: 212-633-3820; E-mail: reprints@elsevier.com.

*Sleep Medicine Clinics* is covered in *MEDLINE/PubMed (Index Medicus).*

# SLEEP MEDICINE CLINICS

---

### SERIES OF RELATED INTEREST

*Otolaryngologic Clinics of North America*
Available at: https://www.oto.theclinics.com/
*Clinics in Chest Medicine*
Available at: https://www.chestmed.theclinics.com/
*Anesthesiology Clinics*
Available at: https://www.anesthesiology.theclinics.com/

---

**THE CLINICS ARE AVAILABLE ONLINE!**
Access your subscription at:
www.theclinics.com

# Contributors

## CONSULTING EDITORS

**TEOFILO LEE-CHIONG Jr, MD**
Professor of Medicine, National Jewish Health, Professor of Medicine, University of Colorado, Denver, Colorado, USA; Chief Medical Liaison, Philips Respironics, Murrysville, Pennsylvania, USA

**ANA C. KRIEGER, MD, MPH, FCCP, FAASM**
Chief, Division of Sleep Neurology, Medical, Director, Weill Cornell Center for Sleep Medicine, Professor of Clinical Medicine, Professor of Medicine in Neurology and Genetic Medicine, Weill Cornell Medical College, Cornell University, New York, New York, USA

## EDITOR

**MATTHEW R. EBBEN, PhD**
Associate Professor, Center for Sleep Medicine, Weill Cornell Medical College, New York, New York, USA

## AUTHORS

**DANIEL A. BARONE, MD, FAASM, FANA**
Associate Medical Director, Weill Cornell Center for Sleep Medicine, Associate Professor of Clinical Neurology, Weill Cornell Medicine | NewYork-Presbyterian, New York, New York, USA

**MARTHA E. BILLINGS, MD, MSc**
Division of Pulmonary, Critical Care & Sleep Medicine, Department of Medicine, University of Washington School of Medicine, Associate Professor of Medicine, UW Medicine Sleep Center, Harborview Medical Center, Seattle, Washington, USA

**MEGAN CRAWFORD, PhD**
School of Psychological Sciences and Health, University of Strathclyde, Glasgow, United Kingdom

**STEVEN H. FEINSILVER, MD**
Director, Center for Sleep Medicine, Lenox Hill Hospital, New York, New York, USA; Hope Healthcare, Hamilton, Bermuda; Professor of Medicine, Zucker School of Medicine at Hofstra Northwell, New York, New York, USA

**MARIANA DELGADO FERNANDES, MD**
Laboratorio do Sono, Instituto do Coracao (InCor), LIM 63, Divisão de Pneumologia, Hospital das Clinicas HCFMUSP, Faculdade de Medicina, Universidade de São Paulo, São Paulo, São Paulo, Brazil

**PEDRO R. GENTA, MD**
Laboratorio do Sono, Instituto do Coracao (InCor), LIM 63, Divisão de Pneumologia, Hospital das Clinicas HCFMUSP, Faculdade de Medicina, Universidade de São Paulo, São Paulo, São Paulo, Brazil

**MARTA KAMINSKA, MD, MSC**
Respiratory Epidemiology and Clinical Research Unit, Research Institute of the McGill University Health Centre–Montreal, Respiratory Division & Sleep Laboratory, McGill University Health Centre–Montreal, Montreal, Quebec, Canada

**LEON LACK, PhD**
Adelaide Institute for Sleep Health, FHMRI Sleep Health, College of Education, Psychology and Social Work, Flinders University, Bedford Park, Australia

**ANNIE C. LAJOIE, MD**
Respiratory Epidemiology and Clinical
Research Unit, Research Institute of the McGill
University Health Centre–Montreal, Montréal,
Quebec, Canada

**JEANE LIMA DE ANDRADE XAVIER, PT**
Laboratorio do Sono, Instituto do Coracao
(InCor), LIM 63, Divisão de Pneumologia,
Hospital das Clinicas HCFMUSP, Faculdade
de Medicina, Universidade de São Paulo, São
Paulo, São Paulo, Brazil

**GERALDO LORENZI-FILHO, MD**
Laboratorio do Sono, Instituto do Coracao
(InCor), LIM 63, Divisão de Pneumologia,
Hospital das Clinicas HCFMUSP, Faculdade
de Medicina, Universidade de São Paulo, São
Paulo, São Paulo, Brazil

**ANNA M. MAY, MD, MS**
Research Section and Sleep Section, VA
Northeast Ohio Healthcare System, Research
K116, Louis Stokes Cleveland VAMC,
Assistant Professor of Medicine, Division of
Pulmonary, Critical Care, and Sleep Medicine,
Department of Medicine, Case Western
Reserve University, Cleveland, Ohio, USA

**TEMITAYO OYEGBILE-CHIDI, MD, PhD,
FAAN**
Associate Clinical Professor, Pediatric
Neurology, Epilepsy and Sleep Medicine,
Department of Neurology, UC Davis School of
Medicine, MIND Institute, Center for Mind and
Brain, University of California, Davis,
Sacramento, California, USA

**LISA RAVDIN, PhD, ABPP**
Associate Professor, Department of
Neurology, Weill Cornell Medicine, New York,
New York, USA

**ALAN Z. SEGAL, MD**
Associate Professor of Clinical Neurology,
Weill Cornell Medicine | NewYork-
Presbyterian, New York, New York, USA

**NITIN K. SETHI, MD, MBBS, FAAN**
Associate Professor, Department of
Neurology, NewYork-Presbyterian Hospital,
Weill Cornell Medical Center, New York, New
York, USA

**ALEXANDER SWEETMAN, PhD**
Adelaide Institute for Sleep Health, FHMRI
Sleep Health, College of Medicine and Public
Health, Flinders University, Bedford Park,
Australia

**MICHELLE VARDANIAN, M.Phil**
Department of Applied Psychology, New York
University, York, New York, USA

**DOUGLAS M. WALLACE, MD**
Department of Neurology, Sleep Medicine
Division, University of Miami Miller
School of Medicine, Neurology Service,
Bruce W. Carter Department of Veterans
Affairs Medical Center, Miami, Florida,
USA

**TERRI E. WEAVER, PhD, RN, ATSF, FAASM**
Dean Emerita, Professor Emerita of
Biobehavioral Nursing Science, College of
Nursing, University of Illinois Chicago,
Chicago, Illinois, USA; Professor Emerita,
School of Nursing, University of
Pennsylvania, Philadelphia, Pennsylvania,
USA

**JEREMY A. WEINGARTEN, MD, MBA, MS**
Associate Professor of Clinical Medicine, Weill
Cornell Medical College, New York, New York,
USA; NewYork-Presbyterian Brooklyn
Methodist Hospital, Brooklyn, New York,
USA

# Contents

> Although data are limited, studies suggest on average lower positive airway pressure use in Black, indigenous, and people of color (BIPOC) compared with Whites in most but not all studies. Most of these observational studies are certainly limited by confounding by socioeconomic status and other unmeasured factors that likely contribute to differences. The etiology of these observed disparities is likely multi-factorial, due in part to financial limitations, differences in sleep opportunity, poor sleep quality due to environmental disruptions, and so forth. These disparities in sleep health are likely related to chronic inequities, including experiences of racism, neighborhood features, structural, and contextual factors. Dedicated studies focusing on understanding adherence in BIPOC are lacking. Further research is needed to understand determinants of PAP use in BIPOC subjects and identify feasible interventions to improve sleep health and reduce sleep apnea treatment disparities.

> Obstructive sleep apnea is one of the most common chronic respiratory illnesses, causing daytime sleepiness and cognitive and cardiovascular morbidity. The most successful treatment has been with positive airway pressure (continuous positive airway pressure or bilevel positive airway pressure). It has been surprisingly difficult to demonstrate improvement in these outcomes with continuous positive airway pressure treatment. This may be because of difficulty quantifying the illness, and heterogeneity in pathophysiology and clinical presentations. This article reviews what has been proven about clinical outcomes, and what is likely if not completely proven.

> Obstructive sleep apnea (OSA) is a common disorder that is increasing in prevalence, both in the United States and worldwide. Continuous positive airway pressure (CPAP), the gold-standard treatment for OSA, is cost-effective from both a payer and societal perspective. Alternative treatments of OSA, including oral appliance therapy, various surgeries, and hypoglossal nerve stimulation have also been evaluated from a cost-effectiveness perspective although results are less consistent. Some studies directly compare these alternative therapies with CPAP. This review will discuss the available literature for cost-effectiveness analysis in the treatment of OSA.

Continuous positive airway pressure is the gold standard treatment for obstructive sleep apnea. Different interfaces with distinct characteristics, advantages, and disadvantages are available, which may influence long-term adherence. Oronasal masks have been increasingly used. However, recent evidence suggest that nasal masks are more effective when continuous positive airway pressure is used to treat obstructive sleep apnea. The main objective of this review is to describe the basis for the selection of the interface for the treatment of obstructive sleep apnea with continuous positive airway pressure.

The treatment of chronic hypoventilation usually requires noninvasive ventilation. However, upper airway obstruction can lead to hypoventilation in conditions such as obesity-hypoventilation syndrome, or chronic obstructive lung diseases (overlap syndrome). In these situations, continuous positive airway pressure can be an effective therapeutic option. This article reviews the pathophysiology of sleep-related hypoventilation, discusses situations where treatment with continuous positive airway pressure is feasible and briefly outlines noninvasive ventilation modes and settings for the treatment of common sleep-related hypoventilation disorders.

About half of continuous positive airway pressure (CPAP)-treated patients are adherent, substantially affecting efficacy. A limitation to understanding predictors of adherence is the lack of a singular definition. Univariate analyses have suggested an array of factors that are statistically significant and reflect disease pathophysiology, clinical features, demographic characteristics, device-related variables, and psychological factors, but whether differences are clinically meaningful is unclear. There have been limited applications of multiple regression to compare the relative influence of multiple variables. This review article considers categories of variables that have been explored and suggests those that may be labeled "best" predictors in understanding CPAP use.

Comorbid insomnia and sleep apnea (COMISA) is a highly prevalent and debilitating condition that is more difficult to treat compared with insomnia alone or sleep apnea alone. Approximately 30% to 50% of sleep clinic patients with sleep apnea report comorbid insomnia symptoms. Comorbid insomnia is associated with lower adherence to positive airway pressure therapy for obstructive sleep apnea. Management approaches that include targeted treatments for both insomnia and sleep apnea lead to the best treatment outcomes for patients with COMISA. Therefore, sleep clinics should incorporate insomnia and COMISA management pathways including access to cognitive behavioral therapy for insomnia.

Obstructive sleep apnea (OSA) is characterized by repetitive episodes of complete or partial upper airway obstruction during sleep, with a worldwide estimate of 936 million sufferers. Treatments of OSA include continuous positive airway pressure (CPAP), weight loss, positional therapy, oral appliances, positive upper airway pressure, oro-maxillofacial surgery, hypoglossal nerve stimulation, and bariatric surgery, and others, with CPAP being the most commonly prescribed treatment. In this review, the neurologic conditions of stroke, cognitive decline, epilepsy, and migraines will be discussed as they relate to OSA. Additionally, the literature regarding improvement in these conditions following treatment with CPAP will be explored.

Pediatric obstructive sleep apnea is becoming more common and better diagnosed and treated. It is seen in children with obesity, genetic disorders, neuromuscular disorders, and congenital malformations. After adenotonsillectomy, continuous positive airway pressure (CPAP) is a major mode of treatment. CPAP is traditionally initiated by titrating in the laboratory. However, auto-CPAP titration in the home environment is becoming more adopted as an option. When children are adherent to CPAP, there are significant benefits to treatment, both short-term and long-term. The short-term benefits include improved behavior, focus, attention, and improved sleep. The long-term benefits include improved cardiovascular and metabolic comorbidities.

Both epilepsy and obstructive sleep apnea are common conditions and hence frequently coexist in a given patient. A complex bidirectional relationship exists between the 2 conditions where the presence of one affects the other. Treatment of obstructive sleep apnea with continuous positive airway pressure may improve seizure control in medically refractory epilepsy patients, leading to improved quality of life. Understanding of this complex relationship between epilepsy, sleep, and sleep disorders such as obstructive sleep apnea continues to evolve.

Obstructive sleep apnea (OSA) is highly prevalent sleep disorders that disrupt sleep through fragmentation, frequent awakenings, and intermittent hypoxia. Both OSA and cognitive decline increase in prevalence with factors such as increasing age and body mass. Multiple areas of cognition can be affected, including attention, executive function, memory, as well as emotional functioning through direct effects on brain health. Although positive airway pressure therapy has shown to improve some aspects of cognitive functioning, it does not fully alleviate all cognitive complaints. Inclusion of complementary approaches to combat these complaints with OSA could potentially enhance treatment outcomes.

# Preface

# Continuous Positive Airway Pressure Therapy for Sleep Apnea: A Newly Controversial Topic

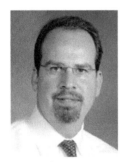

Matthew R. Ebben, PhD
*Editor*

Until recently, treatment for obstructive sleep apnea (OSA) was not a controversial topic. Untreated OSA is associated with increased rate of myocardial infarction, stroke, hyperlipidemia, hypertension, diabetes, and arrhythmias, including atrial fibrillation and pulmonary hypertension, to mention just a few of its most significant associated conditions. Because continuous positive airway pressure (CPAP) is a safe and effective treatment to reduce sleep apnea, it has been assumed for decades to reduce associated cardiovascular risks. Nonetheless, recent empirical data have not, overall, confirmed the benefits of sleep apnea treatment for cardiovascular health. This has understandably shocked the field of sleep medicine, which as a collective whole has been a strong advocate for the benefits of OSA treatment on cardiovascular well-being.

Many have speculated on why studies on CPAP have not confirmed the expected benefits; some cite lack of treatment compliance, and others suggest that the apnea hypopnea index is an imperfect measure of apnea (although CPAP treatment appears to benefit nearly all methods that have been proposed to measure OSA). Nonetheless, considering our current knowledge, many of the supposed benefits can no longer be presumed. However, it's important not to overlook the benefits that have been associated with CPAP use,

particularly daytime alertness, and possibly improved blood pressure. Treatment of these issues alone can significantly improve quality of life for patients and should not be diminished or overlooked. Therefore, CPAP has great value to public health and safely and should continue to be strongly promoted as a treatment for apnea.

The collection of articles in this issue of *Sleep Medicine Clinics* takes a comprehensive look at many aspects of sleep apnea treatment. Topics range from reviews of the outcome data of CPAP treatment in diverse populations, to practical analysis of different mask interfaces, and how to treat hypoventilation with positive airway pressure. Like the field, authors of various articles discuss many of the same research studies, but often with different and sometimes opposing views, particularly when discussing the benefits or lack thereof of CPAP on cardiovascular risks. This makes for interesting reading.

Matthew R. Ebben, PhD
Center for Sleep Medicine
Weill Cornell Medical College
425 East 61st Street, 5th Floor
New York, NY 10065, USA

*E-mail address:*
mae2001@med.cornell.edu

Sleep Med Clin 17 (2022) xi
https://doi.org/10.1016/j.jsmc.2022.09.007
1556-407X/22/© 2022 Published by Elsevier Inc.

# Racial Differences in Positive Airway Pressure Adherence in the Treatment of Sleep Apnea

Anna M. May, MD, MS[a,b,*], Martha E. Billings, MD, MSc[c]

## KEYWORDS

• Racism • Segregation • Neighborhood environment • CPAP Adherence • Sleep apnea • Disparities

## KEY POINTS

• Positive airway pressure (PAP) use differs by race and ethnicity with lower adherence more often in non-white subjects.
• Several factors contribute to lower adherence including the residential environment, socioeconomics, and structural racism.
• Systemic racism has led to lower neighborhood quality and lower socioeconomic position for non-white people.
• Systemic and targeted racism decrease the ability to get appropriate health care assistance to improve positive airway pressure adherence.

## POSITIVE AIRWAY PRESSURE ADHERENCE DISPARITIES: DIFFERENCES BY RACE/ ETHNICITY

Positive airway pressure (PAP) is an effective treatment of sleep apnea, but consistent use has plagued this therapy since inception. While overall adherence has improved with advances in PAP technology, masks, and tele-monitoring, these adherence gains have not been uniform across racial and ethnic groups. Observational studies and clinical trials have noted differences in PAP adherence by race and ethnicity, with lower utilization of PAP therapy in non-white participants. Determinants of PAP utilization habits are complex and multifactorial (**Fig. 1**). However, some of the differences observed by race and ethnicity are related to systemic societal constructs and contextual issues.[1] Chronic discrimination and racism, racialized segregation, and the resulting decline of the built and social environment impacts sleep[2] — regularity, opportunity, duration, and quality. The resulting sleep disparities likely affect PAP use.

### Positive Airway Pressure Use Differences by Race/Ethnicity

Randomized trials to observational studies data show consistent disparities with more hours of PAP use in white versus non-white participants. A multi-center randomized trial comparing home study versus full polysomnography diagnostic and treatment pathways, published in 2011, found

The authors have no conflicts of interest to disclose.
[a] Research Section and Sleep Section, VA Northeast Ohio Healthcare System, Cleveland, OH, USA; [b] Division of Pulmonary, Critical Care, and Sleep Medicine, Department of Medicine, Case Western Reserve University School of Medicine, Cleveland, OH, USA; [c] Division of Pulmonary, Critical Care & Sleep Medicine, Department of Medicine, University of Washington School of Medicine, UW Medicine Sleep Center, Harborview Medical Center, Box 359803, 325 Ninth Avenue, Seattle, WA 98104, USA
* Corresponding author. Research K116, Louis Stokes Cleveland Medical Center, 10701 East Boulevard, Cleveland, OH 44106.
E-mail address: drannamay@gmail.com

| Abbreviations | |
|---|---|
| AASM | American Academy of Sleep Medicine |
| BIPOC | Black, Indigenous, and people of color |
| CMS | Centers for Medicare and Medicaid Services |
| COPD | Chronic obstructive pulmonary disease |
| CPAP | continuous positive airway pressure |
| DME | durable medical equipment |
| PAP | positive airway pressure |
| SES | socioeconomic status |
| US | United States of America |
| VA | Department of Veterans Affairs |

large differences were observed by race, with 92 min/d less PAP use among Black participants compared with whites.[3] In a sham versus active PAP randomized trial, the white race was associated with greater adherence in adjusted analysis by 75 min/d, more so in women.[4] An observational study in Chicago also found a mean 56 min/d lower adherence in Black participants compared with white participants.[5] PAP adherence was lower in Black participants compared with white across 73% of observational studies in the United States (US).[6]

Observational studies from veteran affairs (VA) have offered a window into comparing adherence among Veterans by race, with similar PAP coverage within the integrated health system. In a single-center study in Miami of a diverse cohort of predominantly men, Black participants had a mean of 1.6 hour less continuous PAP (CPAP) use than white subjects. In adjusted analysis, Black race remained associated with adherence although this was not adjusted by socioeconomic status (SES).[7] A similar study of Veterans in Tampa found similar differences by race, with black Veterans half as likely as white Veterans to use CPAP.[8] This difference by race was not observed in a 2009 study of Philadelphia Veterans variations in CPAP use by neighborhood socio-economic status were noted.[9] Philadelphia is a highly segregated city with the lowest SES, most disadvantaged neighborhoods being predominantly black residents, which may have limited adjustment.[10] A more recent VA study in Los Angeles (a less segregated city with declining segregation by 2000) showed differences in adherence by race, with lower odds of reaching Centers for Medicare and Medicaid Services (CMS) adherence among Black veterans compared with others after adjusting for neighborhood SES.[11] Veterans are more often male and in lower SES yet have no limitations on PAP device and supply coverage compared with those relying on Medicare or private insurance. The pattern of lower adherence in black and low SES neighborhood Veterans suggests an underlying systemic etiology.

## Systemic Racism and Discrimination

The sleep health disparities may be partly attributed to the effects of systemic racism and white supremacy. Black, indigenous, and people of

### Potential Contributors to Disparities in PAP Adherence

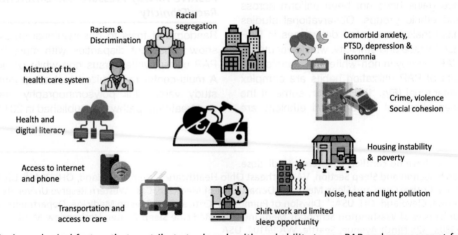

**Fig. 1.** Socio-ecological factors that contribute to sleep health and ability to use PAP and may account for differences by race and ethnicity in PAP adherence. The factors include 1. Societal – racial segregation, racism, discrimination; 2. Neighborhood – crime, heat pollution, social cohesion; 3. Access – transportation, digital literacy, internet; 4. Individual – limited sleep opportunity, anxiety, insomnia, and mistrust. (Icons obtained from flaticon.com.)

color (BIPOC) have suffered the legacy of enslavement, European colonialism, and genocide and the intergenerational trauma remains.[12] Discrimination and political oppression over generations and across the lifespan have marked health consequences. Racism has been endemic to medicine historically, fostering prejudice and stereotypes in health care.[13] BIPOC people have worse health outcomes from infant mortality to dementia in the US.[13] Sleep health is similarly worse in BIPOC with lower sleep quality, underdiagnosis, and undertreatment of sleep disorders.[14]

Implicit bias can impact medical decision-making and quality of care.[15] These implicit biases may negatively influence interactions with sleep providers and durable medical equipment (DME) company staff when non-white individuals struggle with PAP use. Cultural competency and sensitivity are necessary to build rapport and foster patient–provider relationships to enhance adherence.[16] Additionally, the lack of diverse sleep provider workforce may lead to more patient–provider discordance and less resulting trust and a weaker alliance. Data from the American Academy of Sleep Medicine (AASM) Diversity Equity and Inclusion committee show that under-represented minorities make up less than 20% of AASM membership, specifically only 3% Black and 6% Hispanic/Latinx AASM members (although reporting of race/ethnicity was low at 31%).[17] Sleep medicine would benefit from recruiting BIPOC providers, improving diversity and creating a workforce representative of the communities and populations they serve. While concordance has not been studied in PAP adherence, studies of adherence to cardiovascular medications suggest that patient–provider concordance, as well as communication, is associated with better adherence.[18,19]

Discrimination by race and ethnicity additionally can lead to insomnia and poor sleep. Perceived discrimination has been associated with sleep problems and mediates differences in sleep by race. In the Sister Study, those reporting discrimination had higher rates of insomnia symptoms and short sleep duration.[20] Chronic discrimination in the form of microaggressions, stereotype threats can serve as external threats and impair the ability to be vulnerable in sleep.[21] Active discrimination against Hispanics at both a structural level and at an individual, everyday level (so-called microaggressions) increase stress which adversely impacts sleep.[22] Those experiencing racism may have lower quality sleep due to greater "racism-related" vigilance—an inability to set aside worry and stress due to lifelong experiences with discrimination. A survey study of 3000 Chicago residents found that racism-related vigilance mediated the association of difficulty falling asleep or maintaining sleep with the Black race.[23] These lived experiences of oppression and racism that result in poor sleep, insomnia, and shorter sleep may contribute to lower PAP use and less PAP adherence as a result.

### Racialized Segregation

Racialized residential segregation due to historical housing policies has contributed to inequities. Federal government loans were not granted for home mortgages in "redlined" communities, flagged as higher risk investment properties due in part to large black populations. These neighborhoods were outlined by red lines on maps of 239 US cities by the Home Owner's Loan Corporation staff. Additional racially restrictive covenants in housing deeds and community associations barred black home ownership in cities throughout the US.[12] The consequences of this state-sanctioned racism are higher rates of poverty, unemployment, and low home ownership in non-white communities, due to the chronic economic and social deprivation of these areas.[24] This segregation has long-lasting health impacts as neighborhood has been associated with cardiovascular health, cancer risk and outcomes and infectious diseases such as tuberculosis and SARS-CoV2 pandemic.[25] Racialized segregation has also been associated with PAP use. Recent real-world data gathered from a large nationwide sample (80,000 individuals) investigated if PAP use differed by neighborhood segregation rates. The study identified differences in PAP adherence to the racial composition of neighborhoods. PAP users residing in areas with a high proportion of Black or Hispanic residents had 2% lower rates of meeting CMS PAP adherence requirements compared with those neighborhoods with few non-white residents. PAP users residing in communities with greater than 25% Black or Hispanic residents in their neighborhood averaged 22 fewer minutes than those with less than 1% Black or Hispanic neighborhood composition.[26] While this study is limited in its ability to adjust for individual factors, it illustrates the association of racialized segregation with sleep health at the neighborhood level.

### Sleep Duration

On average, BIPOC community members have a shorter sleep duration, increased sleep fragmentation, and lower slow-wave sleep than the white community in surveyed US population.[27] When assessed as a categorical variable, more Black individuals were more likely to be short sleepers ($\leq$6 hours/night) compared with non-Hispanic whites individuals.[28,29] In addition, when this is examined more granularly, Black Americans have 2.5 the odds of habitually sleeping less than 5 hours a night and twice the odds of sleeping between 5 and 6 hours/night. Asian and non-Mexican Hispanic Americans had 2 to 3 times the odds of sleeping less than 5 hours/night.[30] Data from the National Health Interview Survey reveal that compared with white Americans, Black and Native Hawaiian/Pacific Islanders report sleeping less than 7 hours per night.[31] The determinants of these differences in sleep are multifactorial, but likely related to socio-ecological factors.[32]

Time asleep affects PAP adherence: those with less sleep opportunity will have less PAP use. Adequate adherence for continued payer coverage of PAP requires 4 hours of use for at least 70% of nights. This metric does not account for differences in sleep duration.[33,34] This is borne out by a secondary analysis of the HomePAP trial, which found decreased sleep duration and increased sleep latency mediated the association of black race with PAP adherence.[33] Studies suggest that Hispanic individuals also have shorter sleep time compared with white individuals.[35] Therefore, people living in marginalized communities may have a harder time meeting the adherence threshold than comparable nonmarginalized communities. Accounting for shorter total sleep duration, PAP use as a proportion of sleep time may not be as different by race or ethnicity.

### Built Environment

The structure of a neighborhood can significantly affect how people use it. The built environment encompasses all of the different physical structures and amenities of a neighborhood including buildings, sidewalks, bike lanes, parks, food store availability, restaurants, and recreational facilities. The built environment also influences ambient exposures in the neighborhood, such as traffic noise, air pollution, and inopportune light. Disparities in neighborhood exposures and amenities are secondary to long-term structural and institutional forces leading to racial segregation as referenced above. The neighborhood features have a strong influence on sleep duration, quality, and timing. They may also influence the risk of underlying sleep apnea.[36] Through the effects on sleep, these neighborhood features may impact PAP adherence.

Neighborhood geographic characteristics such as greenness versus urban blight contributes to different sleep patterns. Prior observational work suggests that neighborhoods with more tree canopy, water features, and green space have higher average sleep time.[37] Neighborhood greenness is also associated with decreased perceived stress and cardiovascular disease.[38,39] In contrast, those with neighborhood deprivation—more urban noise, litter, blight, and crime—engender more sleep disturbance and shorter sleep time.[40–43] Some of these factors affect the comfort of the sleeping environment—loud sounds, bright lights shining through windows—making it more difficult to sleep. Other features, like the presence of litter and abandoned homes or properties, pose safety hazards and increase stress over possible ne'er-do-wells taking up residence or increasing the risk for burglary and other crimes. Crime can make people feel unsafe in their house via 2 mechanisms. First, crime directly decreases sleep by increasing worry about home invasion leading to hypervigilance. The second, posttraumatic stress disorder can develop in some who have been victims of crime. A cardinal feature of this disorder is hypervigilance, insomnia, and nightmares; all of these changes can decrease or disrupt sleep and make PAP use more challenging.

Several studies have linked air pollution with the development of sleep apnea.[44–47] Poor air quality is also associated with chronic pulmonary disease exacerbation, such asthma and chronic obstructive pulmonary disease (COPD), both disorders more prevalent in Black individuals compared with white individuals.[48,49] Exacerbations of these chronic diseases may make wearing PAP difficult because of the discomfort from coughing while on PAP and the increased resistance of the airways during exacerbation making exhaling more difficult. In addition, hospitalizations, if not accounted during adherence checks appropriately can lead to a falsely low measure of adherence (because the days the patient is hospitalized or in the emergency room are counted as them not using PAP). However, a connection between air quality and PAP adherence has not been formally assessed in research studies.

Nonmaterial environmental factors can also affect sleep. Excess heat and noise are particularly detrimental to sleep. The lack of tree canopy in urban neighborhoods whereby racial and ethnic minorities are often clustered means the environment is up to 4.0° higher than shaded high-income streets.[50] Racial segregation due to racist housing policies has led to urban heat disparities.[51,52] With the effects of global warming, these redlined neighborhoods are at risk of being urban heat domes. Stress in the work environment also affects sleep and perceived sleepiness.[53] Animal models show that a noisy environment disturbs sleep and facilitates weight gain, itself a risk factor for OSA development.[54]

Multiple studies suggest that neighborhood characteristics influence PAP adherence. Platt and colleagues evaluated 330 Veterans with newly started on PAP for adherence in a relationship to a composite neighborhood disadvantage index.[9] Even after adjustment for sociodemographic characteristics and medical comorbidities, compared with the least neighborhood disadvantage (95th percentile), those with the lowest socioeconomic neighborhoods (5th percentile) had half the adherence per CMS criteria (62.3% vs 34.1%).[9] Schwartz and colleagues had similar findings after examining 2172 Veterans.[8] When taken together, these studies indicate that neighborhood socioeconomic status is associated with PAP use, likely due to neighborhood features.

### Social Environment

Neighborhood social features include safety, social cohesion, fear of crime, and connectivity. These factors dramatically affect long-term physiologic and psychological stress levels and add to the allostatic load. Long-term stress, whether severe or minor, is detrimental to humans. The chronic activation of the fight or flight system because of this stress causes weathering—the premature aging and dysregulation of cells, tissues, organs, and body systems because of chronic stress. This weathering can be seen in the increased and earlier rates of diseases and overall lower lifespans in marginalized communities. Systemic and daily low-level racism, discrimination, and economic deprivation all contribute to the allostatic load. The social environment also contributes via chronic fear about safety and low social support in the neighborhood leaving less mental bandwidth for other issues, such as wearing PAP and more difficulty sleeping. This decrease in the restorative power of sleep additionally adds worse memory, vigilance, and possible cognitive decline in the long term. In addition, increasing the disease burden can impair PAP adherence. Safe housing conditions are associated with objectively better sleep, higher sleep efficiency, and lower wake after sleep onset by actigraphy. Those living in neighborhoods with lower social cohesion and more violence concerns had shorter sleep and lower quality sleep.[22,55]

### Cultural Attitudes

Cultural beliefs, norms, and community attitudes about sleep and health may differ among racial and ethnic groups. Health beliefs explained 31.8% of the variance in adherence in a study of 77 CPAP-naïve patients.[56] In particular, outcome expectation, risk perception, and functional limitations secondary to sleepiness were the most salient factors.[56] Multiple studies found that Black people had maladaptive beliefs about sleep, which could influence the perception of sleep apnea symptoms, side effects, and benefits of therapy, and tenacity for treatment.[28,34] Initial work suggests that Black people have a different conception of healthy sleep and sleep apnea. Those at high sleep apnea risk had more dysfunctional attitudes and beliefs about sleep.[28] Black women more commonly agreed that sleepiness is a sign of laziness. Maladaptive beliefs and attitudes about sleep were more common in black men at high risk for OSA.[34] This sort of conceptualization of sleepiness transitions it from a symptom of a disorder to a personal failing, which may alter patterns of adherence. Knowledge about sleep apnea symptoms was similar among white and Mexican Americans in San Diego; however, medical knowledge about this disorder is unlikely to be heterogeneous across the US. Minority populations often have an underlying distrust of the medical community. Part of this mistrust is rooted in history and prior unethical experimentation and exploitation. For instance, to study natural disease progression, the Tuskegee syphilis study of Black men withheld the cure to syphilis until 1972 even though penicillin was invented in 1943.[57] This is just the most recent in a slew of immoral biomedical experiments inflicted on the Southern Black populace.[57] Structural racism has led to health disparities and maltreatment of members of the Black community up to this day; personal experiences of subpar medical care underscore the problem is not only the past. These past and present injustices all lead to a fear of exploitation and mistrusting environment toward the medical establishment.

Numerous studies highlight the lower CPAP adherence in Black and Hispanic individuals. However, there are few studies of race-specific attitudes and cultural beliefs related to CPAP therapy. A recent randomized controlled trial explored a culturally and linguistically tailored approach to address barriers to OSA among Black patients in an effort to improve PAP adherence.[58]

## SOCIOECONOMICS AND POSITIVE AIRWAY PRESSURE USE

Sleep health disparities by race/ethnicity are similar to those observed by SES, with lower SES populations sleeping less, with lower quality sleep and less PAP use. Racial and ethnic minorities in the US are unfortunately more often clustered in the lower income and lower education groups, a result of structural racism and oppression as noted above.[59] With less economic resources, navigating PAP device acquisition, maintenance, and coverage requirements is more challenging. Financial barriers to PAP use include greater burden of costs and copays, lack of access to sleep providers, and competing life demands. With less disposable income, many low SES individuals may be unable to obtain extra supplies (eg, ability to purchase an additional mask). Non-white populations may have lower health literacy, language barriers impairing communication with DME companies and health care providers, lack of technology skills, and limited access to internet.[60] Housing instability, a frequent challenge of poverty, has also been associated with lower PAP use.[61] With less resources, other life demands such as work, childcare, household needs may limit available time to focus on sleep apnea treatment. Shift work, more prevalent in non-white and low SES groups, can limit the opportunity to sleep and use PAP.[62] Each of these additional burdens may hinder PAP use and diminish the ability to achieve adherence in these at-risk populations.

## SUMMARY

Although data are limited, studies suggest on average lower PAP use in BIPOC subjects compared with whites in most but not all studies. Most of these observational studies are certainly limited by confounding by SES and other unmeasured factors that likely contribute to differences. The etiology of these observed disparities is likely multifactorial, due in part to financial limitations, differences in sleep opportunity, poor sleep quality due to environmental disruptions, and so forth. These disparities in sleep health are likely related to chronic inequities, including experiences of racism, neighborhood features, structural, and contextual factors. Dedicated studies focusing on understanding adherence in BIPOC are lacking. Further research is needed to understand determinants of PAP use in BIPOC subjects and identify feasible interventions to improve sleep health and reduce sleep apnea treatment disparities.

## FUNDING

This study was supported by Clinical Science Research and Development Career Development Award IK2CX001882 from the United States (U.S.) Department of Veterans Affairs Clinical Sciences Research and Development Service. The funding sources had no role in the design and conduct of the review; interpretation of the data; or the decision to submit the manuscript for publication. he contents of this work do not represent the views of the Department of Veterans Affairs or the United States government.

## CLINICS CARE POINTS

- White OSA patients on average have higher positive airway pressure adherence than non-White OSA patients.
- Racialized segregation has led to neighborhood inequities. Predominantly non-white and lower SES residents are more often living in hotter, noisier, more polluted neighborhoods with less green space and tree canopy.
- Increased under-represented groups in medicine is a moral imperative; lack of diversity impairs care.
- Contextual factors contribute to sleep time and quality and should be assessed during the sleep evaluation as they may impact PAP use.
- Cultural beliefs, normal, and community attitudes towards sleep and sleep apnea may diverge among racial and ethnic groups.
- Education and discussion before starting therapy may prevent therapeutic failure due to lack of use.
- Financial hardship and housing instability may complicate access to and use of positive airway pressure. Alternative sleep apnea therapies may be more appropriate in such patients.

## REFERENCES

1. Williams NJ, Grandne MA, Snipes A, et al. Racial/ethnic disparities in sleep health and health care: importance of the sociocultural context. Sleep health 2015;1:28–35.
2. Johnson DA, Jackson CL, Williams NJ, et al. Are sleep patterns influenced by race/ethnicity - a marker of relative advantage or disadvantage? Evidence to date. Nat Sci Sleep 2019;11:79–95.
3. Billings ME, Auckley D, Benca R, et al. Race and residential socioeconomics as predictors of CPAP adherence. Sleep 2011;34:1653–8.
4. May AM, Gharibeh T, Wang L, et al. CPAP adherence predictors in a randomized trial of moderate-to-severe OSA enriched with women and minorities. Chest 2018;154:567–78.

5. Pamidi S, Knutson KL, Ghods F, et al. The impact of sleep consultation prior to a diagnostic polysomnogram on continuous positive airway pressure adherence. Chest 2012;141:51–7.

6. Wallace DM, Williams NJ, Sawyer AM, et al. Adherence to positive airway pressure treatment among minority populations in the US: a scoping review. Sleep Med Rev 2018;38:56–69.

7. Wallace DM, Shafazand S, Aloia MS, et al. The association of age, insomnia, and self-efficacy with continuous positive airway pressure adherence in black, white, and Hispanic U.S. Veterans. J Clin Sleep Med 2013;9:885–95.

8. Schwartz SW, Sebastião Y, Rosas J, et al. Racial disparity in adherence to positive airway pressure among US veterans. Sleep Breath 2016;20:947–55.

9. Platt AB, Field SH, Asch DA, et al. Neighborhood of residence is associated with daily adherence to CPAP therapy. Sleep 2009;32:799–806.

10. Williams DR, Collins C. Racial residential segregation: a fundamental cause of racial disparities in health. Public Health Rep 2001;116:404–16.

11. Hsu N, Zeidler MR, Ryden AM, et al. Racial disparities in positive airway pressure therapy adherence among veterans with obstructive sleep apnea. J Clin Sleep Med 2020;16(8):1249–54.

12. Bailey ZD, Feldman JM, Bassett MT. How structural racism works - racist policies as a Root cause of U.S. Racial health inequities. N Engl J Med 2021; 384:768–73.

13. Bailey ZD, Krieger N, Agénor M, et al. Structural racism and health inequities in the USA: evidence and interventions. Lancet 2017;389:1453–63.

14. Jackson CL, Redline S, Emmons KM. Sleep as a potential fundamental contributor to cardiovascular health disparities. Annu Rev Public Health 2015;36: 417–40.

15. FitzGerald C, Hurst S. Implicit bias in healthcare professionals: a systematic review. BMC Med Ethics 2017;18:19.

16. Barksdale DJ. Provider factors affecting adherence: cultural competency and sensitivity. Ethn Dis 2009; 19:S5-3-7.

17. 2021 AASM DEI report. Available at: https://aasm.org/about/diversity-and-inclusion/. Accessed October 5, 2021.

18. Schoenthaler A, Allegrante JP, Chaplin W, et al. The effect of patient-provider communication on medication adherence in hypertensive black patients: does race concordance matter? Ann Behav Med 2012; 43:372–82.

19. Traylor AH, Schmittdiel JA, Uratsu CS, et al. Adherence to cardiovascular disease medications: does patient-provider race/ethnicity and language concordance matter? J Gen Intern Med 2010;25:1172–7.

20. Gaston SA, Feinstein L, Slopen N, et al. Everyday and major experiences of racial/ethnic discrimination and sleep health in a multiethnic population of U.S. women: findings from the Sister Study. Sleep Med 2020;71:97–105.

21. Fuller-Rowell TE, Curtis DS, El-Sheikh M, et al. Racial discrimination mediates race differences in sleep problems: a longitudinal analysis. Cultur Divers Ethnic Minor Psychol 2017;23:165–73.

22. Simonelli G, Dudley KA, Weng J, et al. Neighborhood factors as predictors of poor sleep in the Sueno ancillary study of the Hispanic community health study/study of Latinos. Sleep 2017;40.

23. Hicken MT, Lee H, Ailshire J, et al. Every shut eye, ain't sleep"1: the role of racism-related vigilance in racial/ethnic disparities in sleep difficulty. Race Soc Probl 2013;5:100–12.

24. White K, Haas JS, Williams DR. Elucidating the role of place in health care disparities: the example of racial/ethnic residential segregation. Health Serv Res 2012;47:1278–99.

25. White A, Thornton RLJ, Greene JA. Remembering past Lessons about structural racism - Recentering black Theorists of health and society. N Engl J Med 2021;385:850–5.

26. Borker PV, Carmona E, Essien UR, et al. Neighborhoods with greater prevalence of minority residents have lower continuous positive airway pressure adherence. Am J Respir Crit Care Med 2021;204: 339–46.

27. Jackson CL, Powell-Wiley TM, Gaston SA, et al. Racial/ethnic disparities in sleep health and potential interventions among women in the United States. J Womens Health (Larchmt) 2020;29:435–42.

28. Grandner MA, Williams NJ, Knutson KL, et al. Sleep disparity, race/ethnicity, and socioeconomic position. Sleep Med 2016;18:7–18.

29. Adenekan B, Pandey A, McKenzie S, et al. Sleep in America: role of racial/ethnic differences. Sleep Med Rev 2013;17:255–62.

30. Whinnery J, Jackson N, Rattanaumpawan P, et al. Short and long sleep duration associated with race/ethnicity, sociodemographics, and socioeconomic position. Sleep 2014;37:601–11.

31. McElfish PA, Narcisse MR, Selig JP, et al. Effects of race and poverty on sleep duration: analysis of patterns in the 2014 native Hawaiian and pacific Islander national health Interview survey and general national health Interview survey data. J Racial Ethn Health Disparities 2021;8:837–43.

32. Jackson CL. Determinants of racial/ethnic disparities in disordered sleep and obesity. Sleep Health 2017;3:401–15.

33. Billings ME, Rosen CL, Wang R, et al. Is the relationship between race and continuous positive airway pressure adherence mediated by sleep duration? Sleep 2013;36:221–7.

34. Williams NJ, Jean-Louis G, Ceïde ME, et al. Effect of maladaptive beliefs and attitudes about sleep

among community-dwelling African American men at risk for obstructive sleep apnea. J Sleep Disord Ther 2017;6.

35. Loredo JS, Soler X, Bardwell W, et al. Sleep health in U.S. Hispanic population. Sleep 2010;33:962–7.

36. Dong L, Dubowitz T, Haas A, et al. Prevalence and correlates of obstructive sleep apnea in urban-dwelling, low-income, predominantly African-American women. Sleep Med 2020;73:187–95.

37. Johnson BS, Malecki KM, Peppard PE, et al. Exposure to neighborhood green space and sleep: evidence from the Survey of the Health of Wisconsin. Sleep Health 2018;4:413–9.

38. Yeager R, Riggs DW, DeJarnett N, et al. Association between residential greenness and cardiovascular disease risk. J Am Heart Assoc 2018;7: e009117.

39. Pun VC, Manjourides J, Suh HH. Association of neighborhood greenness with self-perceived stress, depression and anxiety symptoms in older U.S adults. Environ Health 2018;17:39.

40. Hale L, Hill TD, Burdette AM. Does sleep quality mediate the association between neighborhood disorder and self-rated physical health? Prev Med 2010;51:275–8.

41. Hale L, Hill TD, Friedman E, et al. Perceived neighborhood quality, sleep quality, and health status: evidence from the Survey of the Health of Wisconsin. Soc Sci Med 2013;79:16–22.

42. Hill TD, Burdette AM, Hale L. Neighborhood disorder, sleep quality, and psychological distress: testing a model of structural amplification. Health Place 2009;15:1006–13.

43. Troxel WM, Haas A, Ghosh-Dastidar B, et al. Broken windows, Broken Zzs: poor housing and neighborhood conditions are associated with objective measures of sleep health. J Urban Health 2020;97: 230–8.

44. Billings ME, Gold D, Szpiro A, et al. The association of ambient air pollution with sleep apnea: the multi-ethnic study of Atherosclerosis. Ann Am Thorac Soc 2019;16:363–70.

45. Lappharat S, Taneepanichskul N, Reutrakul S, et al. Effects of Bedroom environmental conditions on the Severity of obstructive sleep apnea. J Clin Sleep Med 2018;14:565–73.

46. Clark DPQ, Son DB, Bowatte G, et al. The association between traffic-related air pollution and obstructive sleep apnea: a systematic review. Sleep Med Rev 2020;54:101360.

47. Hunter JC, Hayden KM. The association of sleep with neighborhood physical and social environment. Public Health 2018;162:126–34.

48. Ejike CO, Dransfield MT, Hansel NN, et al. Chronic obstructive pulmonary disease in America's black population. Am J Respir Crit Care Med 2019;200: 423–30.

49. Loftus PA, Wise SK. Epidemiology of asthma. Curr Opin Otolaryngol Head Neck Surg 2016;24:245–9.

50. McDonald RI, Biswas T, Sachar C, et al. The tree cover and temperature disparity in US urbanized areas: Quantifying the association with income across 5,723 communities. PLoS One 2021;16: e0249715.

51. Chakraborty T, Hsu A, Manya D, et al. Disproportionately higher exposure to urban heat in lower-income neighborhoods: a multi-city perspective. Environ Res Lett 2019;14:105003.

52. Hoffman JS, Shandas V, Pendleton N. The effects of historical housing policies on resident exposure to Intra-urban heat: a study of 108 US urban areas. Climate 2020;8.

53. Mokarami H, Gharibi V, Kalteh HO, et al. Multiple environmental and psychosocial work risk factors and sleep disturbances. Int Arch Occup Environ Health 2020;93:623–33.

54. Bosquillon de Jenlis A, Del Vecchio F, Delanaud S, et al. Impacts of Subchronic, high-level noise exposure on sleep and metabolic parameters: a Juvenile Rodent model. Environ Health Perspect 2019;127: 57004.

55. Chen-Edinboro LP, Kaufmann CN, Augustinavicius JL, et al. Neighborhood physical disorder, social cohesion, and insomnia: results from participants over age 50 in the Health and Retirement Study. Int Psychogeriatr 2014;1–8.

56. Olsen S, Smith S, Oei T, et al. Health belief model predicts adherence to CPAP before experience with CPAP. Eur Respir J 2008;32:710–7.

57. Gamble VN. Under the shadow of Tuskegee: African Americans and health care. Am J Public Health 1997;87:1773–8.

58. Jean-Louis G, Robbins R, Williams NJ, et al. Tailored Approach to Sleep Health Education (TASHE): a randomized controlled trial of a web-based application. J Clin Sleep Med 2020;16:1331–41.

59. Williams DR, Priest N, Anderson N. Understanding associations between race, socioeconomic status and health: patterns and prospects. Health Psychol 2016;35:407–11.

60. Estacio EV, Whittle R, Protheroe J. The digital divide: examining socio-demographic factors associated with health literacy, access and use of internet to seek health information. J Health Psychol 2019;24: 1668–75.

61. Liou HYS, Kapur VK, Consens F, et al. The effect of sleeping environment and sleeping Location change on positive airway pressure adherence. J Clin Sleep Med 2018;14:1645–52.

62. Reid KJ, Weng J, Ramos AR, et al. Impact of shift work schedules on actigraphy-based measures of sleep in Hispanic workers: results from the Hispanic Community Health Study/Study of Latinos ancillary Sueño study. Sleep 2018;41.

# Outcomes Data for Continuous Positive Airway Pressure Treatment
## What Do We Really Know?

Steven H. Feinsilver, MD[a,b,c],*

## KEYWORDS

- Obstructive sleep apnea • CPAP • Phenotypes • Outcomes

## KEY POINTS

- CPAP remains the most effective way to reduce sleep-related breathing events during sleep.
- Obstructive sleep apnea is a heterogeneous disease with different mechanisms (endotypes) and presentations (phenotypes).
- Apnea-hypopnea index alone is insufficient to describe the disease.
- Outcomes data for CPAP treatment are difficult to interpret because of the heterogeneity of this disease and inadequate and inconsistent descriptions of severity.

Obstructive sleep apnea (OSA) is one of the world's most common chronic respiratory illnesses, affecting perhaps a billion people worldwide.[1] After 40 years of treatment of OSA with continuous positive airway pressure therapy (CPAP) it is clear that this treatment is effective in reducing the number of respiratory events including apneas and hypopneas during sleep. However, it has been more challenging to definitively prove that this treatment improves clinical outcomes. In fact, several large scale clinical trials have been interpreted as failing to show benefit. Possible reasons for this being so challenging are summarized in **Box 1**. This article reviews what has been proven about clinical outcomes, and what is likely if not completely proven.

## IS APNEA-HYPOPNEA INDEX AN APPROPRIATE MEASURE?

OSA is generally defined and quantified by measuring apneas and hypopneas per hour (apnea-hypopnea index [AHI]). This is a convenient measure, but expert based rather than evidence based, and in fact the basic definitions of respiratory events during sleep have changed several times (**Table 1**). Recognizing apnea is straightforward, but hypopneas have had varying definitions including different degrees of oxygen desaturation and respiratory arousals in some standards.[2–5] The current American Academy of Sleep Medicine standards define hypopneas as a 30% reduction in airflow accompanied by a 3% oxygen desaturation or arousal, but permit an alternate definition requiring a 4% desaturation. Unfortunately, many studies of OSA treatment and outcomes do not explicitly state which AHI definition is used. The AHI by itself does not give any information about duration of respiratory events, severity of oxygen desaturations, or sleep quality. Patients with a similar AHI can have different degrees of duration of events and desaturations.[6] The AHI alone does not correlate well with symptoms and signs of sleep apnea.[7] Considering the wealth of data in a polysomnogram, it has been observed that describing this by a single parameter certainly loses a great deal of useful information.[8]

[a] Center for Sleep Medicine, Lenox Hill Hospital, New York, NY, USA; [b] Hope Healthcare, Hamilton, Bermuda; [c] Zucker School of Medicine at Hofstra Northwell, 100 East 77th Street, New York, NY 10075, USA
* Zucker School of Medicine at Hofstra Northwell, 100 East 77th Street, New York, NY 10075.
*E-mail address:* sfeinsil@northwell.edu

Sleep Med Clin 17 (2022) 551–557
https://doi.org/10.1016/j.jsmc.2022.07.010
1556-407X/22/© 2022 Elsevier Inc. All rights reserved.

sleep.theclinics.com

Box 1
Challenges in proving benefit of CPAP

Inconsistent definitions for respiratory events

Reliance on apnea-hypopnea index to define severity

Few randomized clinical trials

Compliance with CPAP often suboptimal

Difficult to blind CPAP trials

Some unattended sleep studies not measuring airflow directly rely on an oxygen desaturation index (ODI), defined as the number of desaturations (3% or 4%) occurring per hour of sleep or recording time. This measure may be less affected by scorer variability but cannot distinguish central from obstructive events or measure any events not associated with desaturations.

The International Classification of Sleep Disorders[9] defines OSA as an AHI of five or more with symptoms of sleepiness, witnessed apnea or snoring, nonrestorative sleep or insomnia symptoms, or comorbidities including hypertension, cognitive difficulties, coronary disease, congestive heart failure, atrial fibrillation, or type 2 diabetes. Diagnosing a disease based on comorbidities may be unique; patients with frequent nocturnal respiratory events but no symptoms of disturbed sleep, patients with severe sleepiness but few events, and patients with few events but comorbid illness all may be diagnosed with OSA and treated with CPAP. Unsurprisingly, they may have different responses to treatment. Generally mild OSA is considered to be AHI 5 to 15, moderate greater than 15 to 30, and severe greater than 30, but this is not generally adjusted for which AHI definition is used, also adding to disparities in the literature.

## ENDOTYPES AND PHENOTYPES

Patients with OSA are heterogeneous with respect to underlying physiologic mechanism (endotype). These endotypes include: crowded upper airway, impaired upper airway muscle function, increased loop gain, and low arousal threshold.[10] More than one endotype may be present in an individual patient. Endotype may predict response to treatment. For example, a low arousal threshold may be associated with a worse response to CPAP therapy.[11] Patients with a higher arousal threshold may have longer events with more severe hypoxemia. A study examining the time spent with reduced oxygen saturation (hypoxic burden) found this to predict cardiovascular mortality in the Sleep Heart Health Study.[12]

OSA has multiple simultaneous effects, including arousals from sleep, sympathetic nervous system activation, intrathoracic pressure changes, and hypoxia-reoxygenation. Each may have clinically deleterious effects, which are expressed to a varying degree in different patients (phenotypes). Ye and colleagues[13] in a study from the Icelandic Sleep Apnoea Cohort, found three clusters of patient types: disturbed sleep, minimally symptomatic, and excessively sleepy (**Table 2**). Group 1 (disturbed sleep) had highest number of complaints of difficulty initiating and maintaining sleep, restless legs, and daytime napping. Group 2 with minimal symptoms had the highest rates of comorbid cardiovascular disease, despite other observations that cardiovascular risk correlates with daytime sleepiness.[14] This may be because those in Group 3 (most symptomatic) have a shorter lag time before treatment, perhaps preventing the onset of cardiovascular complications. Although these three phenotypes would seem to be different groups, there were no significant differences among groups in AHI or measures of oxygenation.

Table 1
Definitions used in respiratory scoring

| Respiratory Scoring Guidelines | Hypopnea Definition | Alternate Definition |
|---|---|---|
| AASM 1999 Chicago criteria[2] | 50% reduction in airflow | 30% reduction in airflow and 3% desaturation or arousal |
| AASM 2007[3] | 30% reduction in airflow and 4% desaturation | 50% reduction in airflow and 3% desaturation or arousal |
| AASM 2012[4] | 30% reduction in airflow and 3% desaturation or arousal | 30% reduction in airflow and 4% desaturation |
| Centers for Medicare and Medicaid Services[5] | 30% reduction in airflow and 4% desaturation | |

*Abbreviation:* AASM, American Academy of Sleep Medicine.

**Table 2**
**Phenotypes in obstructive sleep apnea**

| Phenotype | Features |
|---|---|
| Group 1: Disturbed sleep | Insomnia, restless legs syndrome |
| Group 2: Minimally symptomatic | Comorbid hypertension, cardiovascular disease more likely |
| Group 3: Excessive sleepiness | Most complaints of snoring, apnea |

Although much more research is needed to evaluate sleep apnea endotypes and phenotypes, it is a reasonable assumption that they have an important influence on the effects of treatment, and that a reliance on AHI alone to describe sleep-disordered breathing is inadequate. Reviewing some of the more significant studies assessing the effects of CPAP treatment on cardiovascular disease, cognitive function including sleepiness, preventing cognitive decline, and mortality shows how difficult it is to measure outcomes for the entire group of patients with OSA.

## OUTCOMES STUDIES
### Cardiovascular Outcomes

There have been seven major randomized clinical trials evaluating cardiovascular outcome, summarized in **Table 3**.

Barbe and colleagues[15] randomized subjects less than 70 years old with no cardiovascular or other chronic disease and no daytime sleepiness with AHI greater than or equal to 20 (using 4% desaturations to define hypopnea). This study failed to find a significant reduction in hypertension or cardiovascular events.

Huang and coworkers[16] studied 73 patients with uncontrolled hypertension and coronary disease for 18 to 36 months and showed some improvement in blood pressure control (and sleepiness) but no difference in adverse cardiac events. This was a small and short study.

In the MOSAIC trial[17] 188 subjects were randomized to CPAP or no CPAP for 2 years. OSA was defined as 4% ODI greater than 7.5. Some patients had significant sleepiness but were believed to have "insufficient daytime symptoms... to warrant CPAP therapy." There was a small reduction in cardiovascular events.

The PREDICT trial enrolled older patients newly diagnosed with OSA for a 1-year trial of CPAP versus best supportive care. Patients were significantly sleepy (Epworth Sleepiness Score [ESS] = 9 or greater) with ODI greater than 7.5. CPAP was found to improve sleepiness but not cardiovascular risk factors or events.[18]

The RICCADSA trial[19] enrolled patients without daytime sleepiness with a history of newly revascularized coronary artery disease to CPAP or no CPAP. At a median follow-up of 57 months, there was no change in the primary end point between those assigned to CPAP or no CPAP, but there was an improvement in cardiovascular risk for those who used CPAP greater than or equal to 4 hours/night.

The SAVE study[20] (Sleep Apnea cardioVascular Endpoints) was an international randomized open label trial of CPAP for patients with preexisting cardiovascular disease with sleep apnea (ODI 4% $\geq$12 on home study). Patients with severe daytime sleepiness (ESS >15) or severe hypoxemia were excluded. Follow-up for up to 4 years failed to show improvement in the primary end point of serious cardiovascular events, although sleepiness was improved. Average CPAP use in the treated group was 3.3 hours per night.

The ISAACC study[21] randomized patients within 3 days after diagnosis of an acute coronary syndrome to CPAP or usual care. Patients were not severely sleepy with an ESS less than or equal to 10 and had an AHI greater than or equal to 15. There was no effect on prevention of major cardiovascular events or death.

None of these studies necessarily prove that there is no cardiovascular benefit to treating OSA with CPAP. Most were secondary prevention studies, that is, patients had preexisting cardiovascular disease. There may be greater benefit in preventing primary cardiovascular events. The time scale of these studies, generally a few years or less, may be insufficient to show effects of disease prevention. All studies were limited by CPAP compliance, which remains a major clinical problem, and none were completely blinded or used a sham CPAP control. Patients for all of these studies were selected based on AHI alone, with no consideration to specific sleep apnea endotypes or phenotypes. For example, if "hypoxic burden" predicts cardiovascular disease and mortality from OSA, this would be an appropriate target for CPAP trials aimed at reduced cardiovascular risk.

### Cognitive Outcomes and Sleepiness

Sleepiness is subjectively measured by the ESS, which asks patients their likelihood of falling asleep on a scale of zero to three on each of eight questions. The total score can be 0 to 24, with ESS of seven or less considered normal.[22] Studies

**Table 3**
**Randomized clinical trials of CPAP for cardiovascular outcomes**

| Study | Subjects | AHI[a] | Outcome Measures | Findings |
|---|---|---|---|---|
| Barbe et al, 2012[15] | <70 y old Not sleepy, no CVD | ≥20 (4%) | Cardiovascular events at 4 y | Not significant |
| Huang et al, 2015[16] | Hypertension and CVD | ≥15 (4%) | Blood pressure ESS score | Improved blood pressure control and sleepiness |
| MOSAIC[17] | Insufficient symptoms to warrant CPAP | ODI >7.5 (4%) | Cardiovascular events at 2 y Sleepiness | Minimal improvement in CV events ($P = .049$); sleepiness improved |
| PREDICT[18] | Sleepy (ESS ≥9) 65 or older | ODI ≥7.5 (4%) | ESS score CV risks and events at 1 y | Sleepiness improved, no effect on CV |
| RICCADSA[19] | Not sleepy (ESS <10); coronary disease with revascularization | AHI ≥15 (4%) | CV mortality, MI, new revascularization | Reduced risk in those who used CPAP ≥4 h/night |
| SAVE[20] | Not severely sleepy (ESS <16) | ODI ≥12 (4%) | Cardiac events or death at mean 3.7 y | Primary outcome no effect |
| ISAACC[21] | Acute coronary syndrome, ESS <11 | AHI ≥15 (4%) | Cardiac events at median 3.35 y | No effect |

*Abbreviations:* AHI, apnea-hypopnea index; CPAP, continuous positive airway pressure; CV, cardiovascular; CVD, cardiovascular disease; ESS, Epworth Sleepiness Score; MI, myocardial infarction; ODI, oxygen desaturation index.
[a] % in parentheses denote percent decrease in oxygen saturation used to define hypopneas or desaturation for ODI.

including Antic and colleagues[23] have been able to show improvement in ESS and tests of neurocognitive function after 3 months of CPAP treatment compared with baseline. However, prospective clinical trials comparing CPAP treatment with no treatment have been more difficult to interpret.

Four studies have looked at cognitive outcomes and daytime sleepiness using the ESS and the Mini-Mental State Exam (MMSE) or Trail Making Test B (TMT-B). They are summarized in **Table 4**. The MMSE measures function over six domains of orientation, attention, calculation, recall, language, and motor skills, with a higher score indicating better function.[24] A one- to three-point change is considered a meaningful decline.[25] This test is designed to measure dementia, and may not be as useful in cognitively normal adults. The TMT-B test involves connecting numbers and letters in circles in ascending order, with a lower number of seconds to complete the task indicating better function.[26]

Monasterio and coworkers[27] randomized subjects with "mild" sleep apnea (AHI between 10 and 30 but apnea index <20) without severe sleepiness or cardiac disease to CPAP or no CPAP. Testing included TMT-B, neurocognitive testing,

multiple sleep latency test, and ESS. No significant differences were seen at 6 months between the treated and untreated groups.

In the PREDICT study[18] ESS was significantly reduced with CPAP compared with no treatment at 3 months, but less so at 12 months. Cognitive tests including MMSE and TMT-B were not significantly changed.

In the nonrandomized PROOF study[28] patients at least 65 years old with severe OSA (AHI >30) were treated or not based on "a common decision with their health care practitioner." They were followed for up to 10 years with MMSE and TMT-B and other testing; CPAP compliance was self-reported. The decline in performance was less in the Wechsler Adult Intelligence Scale-3 similarities test (a measure of logical thinking, verbal concept formation, and abstract reasoning) in patients who were treated with CPAP. Overall MME and TMT-B were no different. ESS at study end was not reported.

Wu and colleagues[29] followed subjects with severe OSA (mean AHI of 61) and reported improved Montreal Cognitive Assessment scores in those randomized to treatment with CPAP for 6 months compared with control subjects.

**Table 4**
**Trials to assess cognitive function with CPAP**

| Study | Subjects | AHI | Measures | Findings |
|---|---|---|---|---|
| Monasterio et al, 2001[27] | Absence of severe sleepiness No cardiac disease | AHI 10–30 but AI <20 | ESS, FOSQ, TMT-B at 6 mo | No significant differences |
| PREDICT[18] | ESS ≥9, 65 or older | ODI ≥7.5 | ESS, TMT-B, MMSE | Only ESS significant |
| Crawford-Achour et al, 2015 (PROOF)[28] | 65 or older Nonrandomized | AHI >30 on home testing (3%) | MMSE, TMT-B, ESS at up to 10 y | Single cognitive measure significant; ESS not reported |
| Wu et al, 2016[29] | Mean age 49.6 No compliance data | AHI >15 Mean AHI 61 | MMSE, MoCA at 6 mo | MMSE nonsignificant, MoCA significant vs control subjects |
| APPLES[30] | Mean age 51.5, BMI 32.3%, 65% male Sham CPAP control subjects | AHI >10 (mean 40) | Multiple measures of cognitive function | Only ESS significant vs control subjects |
| Ponce et al, 2019[31] | 70 y old or older | AHI 15–30 | ESS TMT-B Neurocognitive tests | Only ESS significant vs control subjects |

*Abbreviations:* AHI, apnea-hypopnea index; AI, apnea index; BMI, body mass index; CPAP, continuous positive airway pressure; ESS, Epworth Sleepiness Score; FOSQ, functional outcome of sleep questionnaire; MMSE, Mini-Mental State Exam; MoCA, Montreal Cognitive Assessment; ODI, oxygen desaturation index; TMT-B, Trail Making Test part B.

The APPLES trial (Apnea Positive Pressure Long-term Efficacy Study)[30] randomly assigned more than 1000 patients with AHI greater than 10 to CPAP or sham CPAP for 6 months. Mean AHI was 40. Both subjective (ESS) and objective (Maintenance of Wakefulness testing, Mean Sleep Latency) measures of sleepiness improved in the active treatment group, with improvements in a measure of executive functioning at 2 months but not at 6 months.

A recent study by Ponce and coworkers[31] randomized 145 patients 70 years of age or older to CPAP or no CPAP for 3 months. Primary end point of sleepiness (ESS) improved in the treated group. Neurocognitive measures including TMT-B and tests for anxiety and depression did not significantly improve.

In summary, sleepiness seems to improve with CPAP treatment of OSA, but improvements in measures of cognition may be more subtle and difficult to prove.

## Preventing Cognitive Decline

Although it has been difficult to assess the effects of CPAP treatment on cognitive function in the short term, it is certainly plausible that treatment may prevent cognitive decline caused by chronic sleep-disordered breathing. OSA has been associated with increased markers for Alzheimer disease including amyloid-beta and tau.[32] In an analysis of the Alzheimer's Disease Neuroimaging Initiative database of more than 2000 subjects 55 to 90 years of age, Osorio and colleagues[33] showed patients with self-reported sleep-disordered breathing had an earlier onset of minimal cognitive impairment and CPAP treatment seemed to delay the onset of minimal cognitive impairment.

## Preventing Mortality

There have been four randomized clinical trials evaluating all-cause mortality with CPAP treatment, which failed to show a significant effect.[15,19,20,34] In a meta-analysis of nine nonrandomized trials that reported on mortality associated with the use of PAP versus control there was a clinically significant reduction in risk with a risk ratio of 0.40 (95% confidence interval, 0.24–0.69).[35] Overall quality of evidence was considered low.[34]

## SUMMARY: WHAT DO WE REALLY KNOW?

Positive airway pressure therapy for OSA is clearly the most effective and widely used treatment of this disease, reliably reducing sleep-disordered breathing indices to normal for most patients. However, considering how common this disease seems to be, it is of enormous importance to determine who should be treated, which depends on reliable measures of treatment outcomes. For the most part, this information does not exist. There is strongest evidence for an improvement in daytime sleepiness, suggestive evidence for improving or preventing a decline in neurocognitive function, and poor evidence for preventing cardiovascular disease or mortality. Because most members of the sleep medicine community believe that this therapy is of clear benefit, there seems to be a disconnect with what has been proven. A reasonable hypothesis is that OSA is a heterogeneous disease with different etiologies (endotypes) and different presentations (phenotypes); treating all patients with OSA based on AHI alone may obscure the outcomes data.

## CLINICS CARE POINTS

- CPAP treatment improves daytime sleepiness.
- Treatment probably improves cardiac outcomes at least in patients with daytime sleepiness.
- Treatment clearly improves outcome in patients with coexisting atrial fibrillation.
- Increasing data suggest that treatment of sleep apnea may improve cognitive function and likelihood of progression of dementia.

## DISCLOSURE

The author has nothing to disclose.

## REFERENCES

1. Benjafield AV, Ayas NT, Eastwood PR, et al. Estimation of the global prevalence and burden of obstructive sleep apnoea: a literature-based analysis. Lancet Respir Med 2019;7:687–98.
2. Sleep-related breathing disorders in adults: recommendations for syndrome definition and measurement techniques in clinical research. The Report of an American Academy of Sleep Medicine Task Force Sleep. Sleep 1999;22(5):667–89.
3. Iber C, Ancoli-Israel S, Chesson AL Jr, et al. The AASM manual for the scoring of sleep and associated events: rules, terminology and technical specifications. 1st edition. Westchester (IL): American Academy of Sleep Medicine; 2007.
4. Berry RB, Budhiraja R, Gottlieb DJ, et al. Rules for scoring respiratory events in sleep: update of the 2007 AASM Manual for the scoring of sleep and associated events. Deliberations of the sleep apnea definitions task force of the American Academy of Sleep Medicine. J Clin Sleep Med 2012;8(5):597–619.
5. Centers for Medicare and Medicaid Services. Decision memo for continuous positive airway pressure (CPAP) therapy for Obstructive Sleep Apnea (CAG-00093R2). https://www.cms.gov/medicare-coverage-database/details/nca-decision-memo.aspx?NCAId=204.2008. Accessed 24 Aug 2022.
6. Muraja-Murro A, Nurkkala J, Tiihonen P, et al. Total duration of apnea and hypopnea events and average desaturation show significant variation in patients with a similar apnea-hypopnea index. J Med Eng Technol 2012;36(8):393–8.
7. Tam S, Woodson BT, Rotenberg B. Outcome measurements in obstructive sleep apnea: beyond the apnea-hypopnea index. Laryngoscope 2014;124(1):337–43.
8. Naresh M. Punjabi. COUNTERPOINT: is the apnea-hypopnea index the best way to quantify the severity of sleep-disordered breathing? No Chest 2016;149:16–9.
9. Sateia MJ. International classification of sleep disorders-third edition: highlights and modifications. Chest 2014;146(5):1387–94.
10. Malhotra A, Mesarwi O, Pepin JL, et al. Endotypes and phenotypes in obstructive sleep apnea. Curr Opin Pulm Med 2020;26(6):609–14.
11. Zinchuk A, Edwards BA, Jeon S, et al. Prevalence, associated clinical features, and impact on continuous positive airway pressure use of a low respiratory arousal threshold among male United States veterans with obstructive sleep apnea. J Clin Sleep Med 2018;14:809–17.
12. Azarbarzin A, Sands SA, Stone KL, et al. The hypoxic burden of sleep apnoea predicts cardiovascular disease-related mortality: the Osteoporotic Fractures in Men Study and the Sleep Heart Health Study. Eur Heart J 2019;40(14):1149–57.
13. Ye L, Pien GW, Ratcliffe SJ, et al. The different clinical faces of obstructive sleep apnoea: a cluster analysis. Eur Respir J 2014;44:1600–7.
14. Empana JP, Dauvilliers Y, Dartigues JF, et al. Excessive daytime sleepiness is an independent risk indicator for cardiovascular mortality in community-dwelling elderly: the three city study. Stroke 2009;40:1219–24.
15. Barbé F, Durán-Cantolla J, Sánchez-dela-Torre M, et al. Effect of continuous positive airway pressure on the incidence of hypertension and cardiovascular

events in nonsleepy patients with obstructive sleep apnea: a randomized controlled trial. Jama 2012; 307(20):2161–8.

16. Huang Z, Liu Z, Luo Q, et al. Long-term effects of continuous positive airway pressure on blood pressure and prognosis in hypertensive patients with coronary heart disease and obstructive sleep apnea: a randomized controlled trial. Am J Hypertens 2015;28(3):300–6.

17. Turnbull CD, Craig SE, Kohler M, et al. Cardiovascular event rates in the MOSAIC trial: 2-year follow-up data. Thorax 2014;69(10):950.

18. McMillan A, Bratton DJ, Faria R, et al. Continuous positive airway pressure in older people with obstructive sleep apnoea syndrome (PREDICT): a 12-month, multicentre, randomised trial. Lancet Respir Med 2014;2(10):804–12.

19. Peker Y, Glantz H, Eulenburg C, et al. Effect of positive airway pressure on cardiovascular outcomes in coronary artery disease patients with nonsleepy obstructive sleep apnea. The RICCADSA randomized controlled trial. Am J Respir Crit Care Med 2016;194(5):613–20.

20. McEvoy RD, Antic NA, Heeley E, et al. SAVE Investigators and Coordinators. CPAP for prevention of cardiovascular events in obstructive sleep apnea. N Engl J Med 2016;375(10):919–31.

21. Sánchez-de-la-Torre M, Sánchez-de-la-Torre A, Bertran S, et al, Spanish Sleep Network. Effect of obstructive sleep apnoea and its treatment with continuous positive airway pressure on the prevalence of cardiovascular events in patients with acute coronary syndrome (ISAACC study): a randomised controlled trial. Lancet Respir Med 2020;8(4): 359–67.

22. Johns MW. A new method for measuring daytime sleepiness: the Epworth sleepiness scale. Sleep 1991;14(6):540–5.

23. Antic NA, Catcheside P, Buchan C, et al. The effect of CPAP in normalizing daytime sleepiness, quality of life, and neurocognitive function in patients with moderate to severe OSA. SLEEP 2011;34(1):111–9.

24. Folstein MF, Robins LN, Helzer JE. The Mini-Mental state Examination. Arch Gen Psychiatry 1983; 40(7):812.

25. Andrews JS, Desai U, Kirson NY, et al. Disease severity and minimal clinically important differences in clinical outcome assessments for Alzheimer's

disease clinical trials. Alzheimers Dement (N Y) 2019;5:354–63.

26. Ricker JH, Axelrod BN, Houtler BD. Clinical validation of the oral trail making test. Neuropsychiatry Neuropsychol Behav Neurol 1996;9(1):50–3.

27. Monasterio C, Vidal S, Duran J, et al. Effectiveness of continuous positive airway pressure in mild sleep apnea-hypopnea syndrome. Am J Respir Crit Care Med 2001;164(6):939–43.

28. Crawford-Achour E, Dauphinot V, Martin MS, et al. Protective effect of long term CPAP therapy on cognitive performance in elderly patients with severe OSA: the PROOF study. J Clin Sleep Med 2015;11(5):519–24.

29. Wu SQ, Liao QC, Xu XX, et al. Effect of CPAP therapy on C-reactive protein and cognitive impairment in patients with obstructive sleep apnea hypopnea syndrome. Sleep Breath 2016;20(4):1185–92.

30. Kushida CA, Nichols DA, Holmes TH, et al. Effects of continuous positive airway pressure on neurocognitive function in obstructive sleep apnea patients: the Apnea Positive Pressure Long-term Efficacy Study (APPLES). Sleep 2012;35(12):1593–602.

31. Ponce S, Pastor E, Orosa B, et al. On behalf the Sleep Respiratory Disorders Group of the Sociedad Valenciana de Neumología. The role of CPAP treatment in elderly patients with moderate obstructive sleep apnoea: a multicentre randomised controlled trial. Eur Respir J 2019;54(2):1900518.

32. Mullins AE, Kam K, Parekh A, et al. Obstructive sleep apnea and its treatment in aging: effects on Alzheimer's disease biomarkers, cognition, brain structure and neurophysiology. Neurobiol Dis 2020; 145:105054.

33. Osorio RS, Gumb T, Pirraglia E, et al. Sleep-disordered breathing advances cognitive decline in the elderly. Neurology 2015;84(19):1964–71.

34. Parra O, Sanchez-Armengol A, Capote F, et al. Efficacy of continuous positive airway pressure treatment on 5-year survival in patients with ischaemic stroke and obstructive sleep apnea: a randomized controlled trial. J Sleep Res 2015;24(1):47–53.

35. Patil SP, Ayappa IA, Caples SM, et al. Treatment of adult obstructive sleep apnea with positive airway pressure: an American Academy of Sleep Medicine systematic review, meta-analysis, and GRADE assessment. J Clin Sleep Med 2019;15(2):301–34.

# Cost-Effectiveness of Continuous Positive Airway Pressure Therapy Versus Other Treatments of Obstructive Sleep Apnea

Jeremy A. Weingarten, MD, MBA, MS[a,b,]*

## KEYWORDS

- Cost-effectiveness analysis • Obstructive sleep apnea • Continuous positive airway pressure
- Oral appliances • Sleep apnea surgery • Upper airway stimulation

## KEY POINTS

- Cost-effectiveness analysis is essential in understanding the financial implications of various treatments for obstructive sleep apnea (OSA).
- Continuous positive airway pressure (CPAP) is highly cost-effective from a payer perspective and may in fact be economical from a societal perspective (cheaper to society to treat OSA with CPAP than not treat).
- Although less evidence have accumulated, current literature suggests that oral appliance therapy, surgical intervention, and hypoglossal nerve stimulation may be cost-effective in certain populations.

## INTRODUCTION

Obstructive sleep apnea (OSA) is a disorder characterized by repetitive collapse of the upper airway during sleep resulting in frequent awakenings, poor sleep quality, and excessive daytime sleepiness. Cardiometabolic abnormalities are associated with OSA due to intermittent hypoxia, intrathoracic pressure fluctuations, and cyclical sympathetic surges among other mechanisms.[1–3] Clinically, there is strong epidemiologic evidence associating OSA with hypertension, coronary artery disease, cardiac arrhythmias, heart failure, stroke, and insulin resistance. Although randomized controlled trials of treatment of OSA have not definitively demonstrated benefit, methodological issues plagued these studies, whereas the observational data are much more consistent on treatment reducing the severity of comorbid conditions.[4,5] Treatment options include continuous positive airway pressure (CPAP) therapy, oral appliance therapy (OAT), surgery, and lifestyle modification.[3,6] Although treatment modalities vary in effectiveness and cost, the decision to use one modality over another depends on both clinical characteristics of the disease state and patient preference. In general, PAP is recommended as first-line treatment of OSA patients but the range of treatment options leaves open the possibility of alternative therapies. Many of these modalities have been studies in cost-effectiveness research. This article will review the cost-effectiveness of PAP therapy and its alternatives in treating OSA.

OSA is a common disease. The estimated prevalence of clinically significant OSA in the United States during the period 2007 and 2010 was 10% to 12% among men aged 30 to 49 years,

a Department of Medicine, Weill Cornell Medicine, New York, NY 10065, USA; b NewYork-Presbyterian Brooklyn Methodist Hospital, Brooklyn, NY 11215, USA
* 501 Sixth Street, Wesley House Suite 7A, Brooklyn, NY 11215.
E-mail address: jaw9031@nyp.org

Sleep Med Clin 17 (2022) 559–567
https://doi.org/10.1016/j.jsmc.2022.07.003
1556-407X/22/© 2022 Elsevier Inc. All rights reserved.

| Abbreviations | |
|---|---|
| OSA | Obstructive Sleep Apnea |
| OAT | Oral Appliance Therapy |
| CPAP | Continuous Positive Airway Pressure |
| AHI | Apnea Hypopnea Index |
| CVD | Cardiovascular Disease |
| QALY | Quality-Adjusted LIfe Year |
| ICER | Incremental Cost-Effectiveness Ratio |
| DALY | Disability-Adjusted Life Year |
| PPRS | Platopharyngeal Reconstructive Surgery |
| MLS | Multilevel Surgery |
| HNS | Hypoglossal Nerve Stimulation |
| RCT | Randomized Controlled Trials |

17% to 18% among men aged 50 to 70 years, 3% among women aged 30 to 49 years, and 8% to 9% among women aged 50 to 70 years.[7] The global burden of sleep apnea is high and likely to increase over time as populations expand and risk factors for OSA (primarily obesity) increase over time. Based on the available literature and risk-adjusted models, the estimate of worldwide sleep apnea is 936 million people with an apnea-hypopnea index (AHI) 5 events or greater per hour and 425 million people with an AHI of 15 events or greater per hour.[8] In the United States, the authors estimated that 54 million people have mild or greater OSA (AHI $\geq$5 events/h) and 25 million people with moderate or greater OSA (AHI $\geq$15 events/h). This is in line with a report by Frost and Sullivan[9] in which 29 million people are estimated to have mild or greater OSA, with 80% (23.5 million) undiagnosed.

Sleep disorders pose a significant economic burden on health-care systems and society in general. In the most comprehensive evaluation of costs of sleep disorders, including OSA, insomnia, and restless legs syndrome,[10] overall societal costs for these 3 disorders in Australia in 2019 to 2020 was US$35.4 billion. For the subgroup of OSA in this study, health-care system costs, which included hospital and out-of-hospital services, CPAP costs, medical research costs, and costs of treating conditions attributable to OSA (cardiovascular disease [CVD] as well as workplace accident costs), totaled US$376 million. With the addition of other costs, including productivity costs and disability-adjusted life year losses, the total cost for OSA was US$13.1 billion. The greatest contributor to this cost was workplace productivity costs (absenteeism, presenteeism [suboptimal workplace functioning due to illness/injury], reduced employment, and premature mortality), totaling US$2.7 billion. It should be noted that this study focuses on total societal costs, whereas many studies, particularly in the United States, look at costs from a payer or health-care system perspective and often do not consider workplace productivity costs. The economic impact of OSA in the United States was also evaluated recently; in 2015, diagnosed OSA cost US$12.4 billion from a societal perspective, resulting in a per capita cost of US$2105.[9] The most striking finding of this study was that undiagnosed OSA costs 3 times more at a total of US$150 billion and US$6366 per capita. Given these high costs, it is essential that we systematically evaluate cost-effectiveness of various interventions to allow the largest number of patients to benefit from current therapies.

## COST-EFFECTIVENESS ANALYSIS OVERVIEW

A brief review of cost-effectiveness study technique is essential to understand the following discussion. Cost-effectiveness research is but one method of economic evaluation of an intervention.[11] As will be shown in more detail below, cost-effectiveness analysis compares the costs and the effectiveness (usually measured as the quality-adjusted life year [QALY], which considers total years of life gained due to an intervention adjusted for the quality of life in those years) of an intervention to a reference intervention. Cost–benefit analysis assigns a monetary value to both cost and effectiveness that relies on valuing suffering in terms of dollars, which is difficult to do. Finally, cost-minimization studies evaluate which of 2 interventions, which have proven equivalent effectiveness, costs less.

The fundamental unit of analysis for a cost-effectiveness analysis is the incremental cost-effectiveness ratio (ICER), which can be represented as follows:

$$ICER = \frac{Cost2 - Cost1}{Effect2 - Effect1}$$

where cost of the new intervention (Cost2) is compared with the reference intervention (Cost1), and similarly the effects of new versus referent interventions are compared (Effect2 and Effect1). The variables used for cost and effect depend on the perspective from which the analysis is being undertaken. When determining costs for example, if the analysis is undertaken from a payer's perspective, then direct and indirect medical costs, including the effect of the intervention on downstream comorbid conditions, will be used, whereas the effect on workplace productivity costs will not be included because they do not affect the costs an insurer would incur. Other perspectives include societal, health system, and government perspective.[11] The effect measure can be a specific outcome (ie, reduction in AHI) or more commonly QALYs.

Cost-effectiveness analysis in the literature are frequently 1 of 3 types: trial-based, model-based, or hybrid. Trial-based studies use studies that enroll subjects, model-based studies rely on mathematical models (ie, Markov models), and hybrid studies combine both techniques.[12] There are advantages and disadvantages to the different study types but this is beyond the scope of this article. Three final topics of cost-effectiveness analysis should be mentioned. First, the threshold less than which an intervention is deemed cost-effective is geographically and health-care system based, usually determined empirically by evaluating the prices payers have already paid for certain treatments; in the United States, willingness-to-pay is generally accepted to be US$50,000/QALY, although this is not without controversy.[13] Second, the degree of uncertainty in cost-effective analyses forces researchers to perform extensive sensitivity analyses to properly understand their data and form conclusions.[12] This article will not delve into sensitivity analyses of the discussed studies for brevity. Third, an intervention in which costs are reduced while effectiveness is improved is called "dominant." Although specific costs for the intervention itself may increase (diagnostic testing, medications, devices), downstream savings by reducing costs related to other treatments that may not be needed results in overall negative incremental costs.

## COST-EFFECTIVENESS OF CONTINUOUS POSITIVE AIRWAY PRESSURE

A plethora of studies worldwide have evaluated the cost-effectiveness of CPAP for OSA and found that this treatment modality is cost-effective.[14] Although the studies vary in many respects, in general, with time horizons of at least 5 years, the ICERs are less than the willingness-to-pay threshold. As this article is not a systematic review, this article will focus on studies from the United Kingdom, Canada, the United States, and Australia (**Table 1**). In the United Kingdom, the range of ICERs for CPAP versus no CPAP were −£1845 to £15,337/QALY.[15–19] As stated earlier, a negative ICER is considered "dominant" in that the intervention is cost saving/reducing while also improving effectiveness; this was seen in the ResMed trial[16] and the Guest trial.[19] The only other study that demonstrated a dominant effect was Streatfeild[20] but only from the societal perspective. Most of the UK trials were analyzed from the National Health System perspective and focused primarily on direct costs. The willingness-to-pay in the United Kingdom is generally considered £20,000. In Canada, the range of ICERs for CPAP versus no CPAP was US$2581/QALY to US$7438/QALY from a third-party payer perspective[21–23] and US$314/QALY to US$2167/QALY from a societal perspective,[22,23] which includes productivity losses and other parameters. The ICER for CPAP versus no CPAP in the only study published using US data was US$13,698/QALY.[24] Finally, in a comprehensive study from Australia, which reported effectiveness as disability-adjusted life years (DALYs) averted, the ICER was US$12,495/DALY averted from a health-care system perspective and −US$10,688/DALY averted (a dominant effect) from a societal perspective.[20]

Methodologic differences among the studies reviewed make comparability of these studies difficult. First, different time horizons result in different ICERs; this is because most costs related to CPAP therapy are up-front costs that essentially depreciate over time. Costs for diagnostic sleep studies, initiation and payment for CPAP, and initial follow-up occur in the first 1 to 1.5 years. Changes in the cost of comorbid conditions in the intervention and reference group are most evident several years out from initiation of therapy. The range of ICERs from the UK trials is large, from the dominant (negative) ICERs to more than £15,000/QALY; similarly, the time horizons vary from 12 months to 14 years. The Chilcott and colleagues Trenton Report[18] illustrates the importance of time horizon in evaluating cost-effectiveness studies; from 1 month to 1 year to 2 years to 5 years, the ICER decreases from £99,000 to £8300 to £5200 to £3200/QALY. Most studies looked at a time horizon of 5 years, which is frequently agreed on as the functional life of a CPAP device. However, given that OSA is a

**Table 1**
Cost-effectiveness analyses of continuous positive airway pressure

| Author, Pub Year | Country | Perspective | Time Horizon | Study Design | Base Case | Reference | ICER |
|---|---|---|---|---|---|---|---|
| Touisignant P, 1994 | Canada | Payer | N/A | Trial-based | N/A | No CPAP | US$2581–$7438 |
| Chilcott et al,[18] 2000 | United Kingdom | Payer | 5 y | Model | N/A | No CPAP | £3200 |
| Ayas et al,[22] 2006 | Canada | Payer Societal | 5 y | Model | Mod–sev OSA | No CPAP | US$3354 US$314 |
| Resmed, 2007 | United Kingdom | Payer | 14 y | Model | Sev OSA | No CPAP | –£1620 |
| Guest et al,[19] 2008 | UK | Payer | 14 y | Model | Sev OSA | No CPAP | –£942 |
| Tan et al,[23] 2008 | Canada | Payer Societal | 5 y | Model | Mod–sev OSA | No CPAP | US$2810 US$2167 |
| Sadatsafavi et al,[24] 2009 | United States | Payer | 5 y | Model | Mod–sev OSA | No CPAP | US$13,698 |
| Guest et al,[15] 2014 | United Kingdom | Payer | 5 y | Hybrid | OSA | No CPAP | £15,337 |
| McMillan et al,[17] 2015 | United Kingdom | Payer | 12 mo | Trial-based | OSA | No CPAP | £8750–12,500 |
| Streatfeild et al,[20] 2019 | Australia | Payer Societal | 5 y | Model | Mod–sev OSA | No CPAP | US$12,495 –US$10,688 |

Note: a negative ICER is considered dominant (see text).
*Abbreviations:* N/A, not available; Pub, publication.

lifelong disorder, using shorter time horizons may overestimate the ICER; future cost savings due to improved comorbidities (fewer CVD events and fewer motor vehicle accidents [MVA]) and improved work productivity are not considered.

Another methodologic concern with cost-effectiveness studies of CPAP use in OSA is that there is no agreed on or subscribed to standardization of cost-effectiveness analysis. When an analysis is undertaken from a payer perspective, it is important to realize that different studies use different variables, and that this difference, and the assumptions underlying these different variables, can vastly alter the results of the analysis. If one study looks only at direct medical costs of OSA evaluation and management, including diagnostic testing and CPAP costs, while another also includes cost reduction and QALY improvement related to comorbid condition improvement from adequate OSA therapy, then these studies are evaluating vastly different things. For example, among the reviewed studies performed from a payer perspective, some studies look only at direct medical costs from OSA evaluation and management,[21,22] whereas others analyzed how CVD events and MVA affect the incremental cost of the intervention versus the reference.[16,19] The variability in cost-effectiveness from a societal perspective makes the lack of standardization even more stark; depending on the variables analyzed, ICERs from a societal perspective range from −US$10,688 (dominant) to US$2167/QALY. The differences in ICERs are related to how many variables are included and how costs and QALYs were accounted for. Streatfeild and colleagues[20] performed the most comprehensive analysis by including productivity losses, taxation losses, and welfare costs in addition to extensive clinical costs from CVD, diabetes, and even depression. The more comprehensive the analysis, the closer to the true estimate of the cost-effectiveness of an intervention, although this specificity can also reduce the generalizability of the findings.

## COST-EFFECTIVENESS OF ORAL APPLIANCE THERAPY

Four studies looked at the cost-effectiveness of OAT versus no therapy (**Table 2**)[24–26]; most of these studies looked at patients with mild-to-moderate OSA. In general, OAT was found to be cost-effective at the appropriate willingness-to-pay threshold. In a trial-based, randomized crossover study looking at 3 different types of OAT[25] (a self-molded thermoplastic "boil and bite" appliance (SP1), semi-bespoke appliance in which the patient used dental putty themselves and sent

the mold out for fabrication (SP2), and a fully bespoke/professionally fabricated appliance), all 3 were found to be cost-effective compared with conservative management, although as expected, as the price of the device increases, the ICER also increases (range of −£17,136 [dominant] to £14,876/QALY). The semi-bespoke appliance had the greatest cost-effectiveness, being both cost-saving (dominant) and clinically superior. As discussed above, the time horizon of this study was short at 1 month and therefore calls into question the validity of the findings. Two other studies showed reasonable ICERs for OAT versus no therapy (US$2984 and £6687/QALY); the base case in the first and second studies was moderate-to-severe OSA[24] and mild-to-moderate OSA, respectively,[25] making these 2 studies similar in overall cost-effectiveness while highlighting that in more severe disease, treatment will frequently result in a larger improvement in QALY and thus a lower ICER and increased cost-effectiveness. The final study demonstrated much higher ICERs of €32,976 to €45,579/QALY likely due to evaluating a base case comprising mild-to-moderate OSA in those with low-CVD risk[26]; although the study was more comprehensive by including CVD and MVA in its cost and effectiveness calculations, the low cardiac risk in the base case essentially negates the weight of these events, making the intervention overall less cost-effective.

Several studies compared CPAP therapy with OAT. Three studies looked at direct incremental cost-effectiveness of CPAP versus OAT from a payer perspective. Two of these studies demonstrated good incremental cost-effectiveness of CPAP (where OAT is the reference case) with ICERs of US$27,540 and £15,367/QALY, both well within the willingness to pay threshold.[24,25] This suggests that in patients already using OAT, treating with CPAP instead is cost-effective; although costs may be higher, the improvement in QALY with CPAP versus OAT results in improved cost-effectiveness. These studies looked at base cases of moderate-to-severe OSA and mild-to-moderate OSA respectively without a qualifier as to cardiovascular risk—both included CVD and MVA in their analysis. The third study in which the base case was defined as mild-to-moderate OSA with low cardiovascular risk, the ICERs were extremely high at ~€256,000/QALY[26]; again, as noted above, a low-CV risk in the base case affects the numerator and denominator in the ICER calculation and likely significantly affects both costs and QALY gained from the intervention. A final study directly compared OAT and CPAP (as the reference) from a societal perspective and found that OAT was not cost-effective

**Table 2**
Cost-effectiveness analyses of alternative therapies

| | Author, Pub Year | Country | Perspective | Time Horizon | Study Design | Base Case | Reference | Qualifier | ICER |
|---|---|---|---|---|---|---|---|---|---|
| OAT | Sadatsafavi et al,[24]2009 | United States | Payer | 5 y | Model | Mod-sev OSA | No OAT | | US$2984 |
| | de Vries et al,[27] 2019 | Netherlands | Societal | 12 mo | Trial-based | Mod OSA | CPAP / CPAP | | US$27,540 / €33,701 |
| | Sharples et al,[25] 2014 | United Kingdom | Payer | 1 mo | Trial-based | Mild–mod OSA | No OAT | SP1 / SP2 | −£4117 / −£17,136 |
| | Sharples et al,[25] 2014 | United Kingdom | Payer | Lifetime | Model | Mild–mod OSA | No OAT / CPAP | Bespoke | £14,876 / £6687 / £15,367 |
| | Poullie AI, 2016 | France | Payer | Lifetime | Model | Mild OSA / Mod OSA / Mild OSA / Mod OSA | No OAT / No OAT / CPAP / CPAP | Low-CV risk / Low-CV risk / Low-CV risk / Low-CV risk | €45,579 / €32,976 / €256,048 / €256,278 |
| Surgery | Tan et al,[29] 2015 | United States | Payer | Lifetime | Model | Sev OSA | CPAP / CPAP-PPRS | CPAP-PPRS / CPAP-MLS | US$10,421 / US$84,199 |
| | Kempfle et al,[31] 2017 | United States | Payer | 5/10/15 y | Model | Variable | No Surgery / No Surgery | TR / Septoplasty | Cost-effective / Cost-effective except short-term |
| HNS | Pietzch JB, 2015 | United States | Payer | Lifetime / 10 y | Model | Mod–sev OSA | No HNS | | US$39,471 / US$57,773 |
| | Pietzch JB, 2019 | Germany | Payer | Lifetime / 10 y | Model | Mod–sev OSA | No HNS | | €44,446 / €60,216 |
| | Blissett et al,[37] 2021 | United Kingdom | Payer | Lifetime | Model | Sev OSA | No HNS | | £17,989 |

*Abbreviations:* CV, cardiovascular; Pub, publication; TR, turbinate reduction.

when AHI improvement was the outcome variable (instead of QALY) but was cost-effective when QALY was the outcome variable (ICER of €33,701/QALY, within the willingness-to-pay threshold for the Netherlands).[27]

## COST-EFFECTIVENESS OF SURGICAL INTERVENTION

Surgery as a therapeutic modality is often considered less effective for OSA compared with other modalities in terms of AHI reduction although at times can be more attractive to patients because it is essentially a one-time intervention obviating the nightly use of a CPAP device or oral appliance. In general, surgery is considered an alternate to CPAP or OAT due to the lack of rigorous data demonstrating equivalent efficacy compared with CPAP or OAT.[28] Regardless, cost-effectiveness analysis has been evaluated in both upper airway and nasal surgery (see **Table 2**).

Tan and colleagues[29] evaluated the cost-effectiveness of upper airway surgery compared with CPAP. The authors evaluated both palatopharyngeal reconstructive surgery (PPRS), focusing on uvula-sparing procedures, and multilevel surgery (MLS). In this model-based trial performed from a payer perspective, the base case was a 50-year-old with untreated severe OSA. The incremental costs were evaluated stepwise, first looking at CPAP followed by PPRS and then MLS. CVD, MVA, and surgical complications were included in the analysis. The ICERs of the various strategies were as follows: CPAP versus no treatment was US$3901/QALY, PPRS versus CPAP was US$10,421/QALY, and MLS versus PPRS was US$84,199/QALY. In this analysis, in severe OSA patients intolerant of CPAP, PPRS is a cost-effective treatment while MLS requires a higher willingness-to-pay to be considered cost-effective.

Although nasal surgery is not an effective, corrective therapy in OSA with regards to AHI reduction, it has been found to improve other sleep symptoms such as sleepiness. Often, nasal surgery is performed to improve compliance with CPAP by reducing the required pressure to maintain upper airway patency.[30] Kempfle and colleagues[31] investigated the cost-effectiveness of turbinate reduction and septoplasty as interventions to improve compliance. The study was model-based and varied the base case by low baseline compliance, high baseline compliance, 3-time horizons (5, 10, and 15 years), and a range of costs related to untreated OSA. In their model, the authors assumed that either turbinate reduction or septoplasty improved compliance by 20%. The authors found that turbinate reduction

was cost-effective in all conditions, likely due to its lower surgical costs. Septoplasty was not cost-effective in the group with low baseline CPAP compliance and at shorter time intervals (5 years) but became increasingly cost-effective over longer time horizons.

## COST-EFFECTIVENESS OF HYPOGLOSSAL NERVE STIMULATION

Although a relatively new entrant in the treatment of OSA, hypoglossal nerve stimulation (HNS) has been shown to improve objective and subjective measures in OSA patients with minimal adverse events.[32,33] The main drawback of this intervention is its highly selective nature. Based on the STAR trial data and FDA approval parameters, HNS was initially indicated in the following patients: age 22 years or older, AHI range 20 to 65 events per hour, predominantly obstructive phenotype, no concentric velopharyngeal collapse as assessed on drug-induced sleep endoscopy, absence of other upper airway anatomic findings (tonsillar hypertrophy), and body mass index less than 32 kg/m$^2$. Insurers, including the Center for Medicare and Medicaid Services, have eased indications by including a higher acceptable BMI (<35 kg/m$^2$) and a lower acceptable AHI range (15–65 events per hour).[34]

All studies looking at the cost-effectiveness of HNS were model based, had a lifetime horizon, and added CVD and MVA to its variables (see **Table 2**). Two studies[35,36] by the same investigators evaluated HNS in patients with moderate-to-severe OSA in the United States and Germany. The ICERs of HNS versus no therapy over the lifetime horizon were cost-effective at a willingness-to-pay threshold of US$50,000 and €50,000; the ICER for the US study was US$39,471/QALY and for the German study was €44,446/QALY. When the time horizon was reduced to 10 years, the ICERs were not cost-effective (US$57,773/QALY and €60,216/QALY, respectively). The final study evaluating HNS versus no treatment was performed with a base case of severe OSA intolerant of CPAP therapy.[37] This study had an ICER of £17,989/QALY, again illustrating that as the severity of the base case increases, the presumed effectiveness increases and the ICER decreases. Overall, it seems that HNS is cost-effective particularly looking over a lifetime time horizon, which is appropriate given the chronic nature of OSA.

## SUMMARY

OSA is a chronic disease with significant impact on an individual patient's quality of life, cardiovascular health, and incidence of workplace and traffic accidents. The prevalence of OSA and the likelihood that most patients with OSA are un-diagnosed results in potentially significant strain on health-care economics. It is essential that OSA treatments are evaluated in an economic context for policy decisions. The gold-standard treatment of OSA, namely CPAP, has strong evidence of cost-effectiveness from both a payer and societal perspective. In fact, one model-based study showed that CPAP is cost-saving overall primarily due to its reduction in comorbidity expenses and work productivity losses in the setting of reduced disability-adjusted life years. Alternative modalities for treatment of OSA are also generally cost-effective, including OAT, upper airway and nasal surgery, and HNS, with a few ex-ceptions: although septoplasty and MLS show improved quality-adjusted life years, the overall costs per QALY does not meet the threshold in which payers are likely to be willing to pay. Although recent randomized controlled trials (RCTs) of PAP treatment in OSA such as the SAVE trial[4] did not demonstrate the reductions in cardiovascular morbidity/mortality that were seen in observational and other studies on which the cost-effectiveness analyses are predicated on, there is active debate about the methodology and limitations of these RCTs and their infer-ences.[5,38] Despite these RCTs, the strength and consistency of the evidence of cardiovascular risk reduction in OSA treatment from epidemio-logic studies lends validity to current cost-effectiveness analyses and should be accepted as such until further evidence confirms or refutes the RCT data. Because the prevalence of OSA is only likely to increase given the estimates of currently untreated OSA and the increasing levels of obesity worldwide, further studies are neces-sary to make informed decisions regarding the true cost-effectiveness of different modalities of therapy of OSA.

## CLINICS CARE POINTS

- Evidence supports that CPAP therapy is cost-effective in the treatment of OSAOther trea-ment modalities may be cost-effective in the treatment of OSA in certain patient popula-tions.

## DISCLOSURE

The author has nothing to disclose.

## REFERENCES

1. Bradley TD, Floras JS. Obstructive sleep apnoea and its cardiovascular consequences. Lancet 2009;373(9657):82–93.
2. Dempsey JA, Veasey SC, Morgan BJ, et al. Patho-physiology of sleep apnea. Physiol Rev 2010;90(1):47–112.
3. Veasey SC, Rosen IM. Obstructive sleep apnea in adults. N Engl J Med 2019;380(15):1442–9.
4. McEvoy RD, Antic NA, Heeley E, et al. CPAP for pre-vention of cardiovascular events in obstructive sleep apnea. N Engl J Med 2016;375(10):919–31.
5. Mokhlesi B, Ayas NT. Cardiovascular events in obstructive sleep apnea - can CPAP therapy SAVE lives? N Engl J Med 2016;375(10):994–6.
6. Epstein LJ, Kristo D, Strollo PJ, et al. Clinical guide-line for the evaluation, management and long-term care of obstructive sleep apnea in adults. J Clin Sleep Med 2009;5(3):263–76.
7. Peppard PE, Young T, Barnet JH, et al. Increased prevalence of sleep-disordered breathing in adults. Am J Epidemiol 2013;177(9):1006–14.
8. Benjafield AV, Ayas NT, Eastwood PR, et al. Estima-tion of the global prevalence and burden of obstruc-tive sleep apnoea: a literature-based analysis. Lancet Respir Med 2019;7(8):687–98.
9. Frost & Sullivan. Hidden health crisis costing Amer-ica billions. Underdiagnosing and undertreating obstructive sleep apnea draining healthcare system. 2016.
10. Streatfeild J, Smith J, Mansfield D, et al. The social and economic cost of sleep disorders. Sleep 2021. https://doi.org/10.1093/sleep/zsab132.
11. Muennig P, Bounthavong M. Cost-effectiveness analysis in health : a practical approach. San Fran-cisco, CA: John Wiley & Sons, Incorporated; 2016.
12. Cohen DJ, Reynolds MR. Interpreting the results of cost-effectiveness studies. J Am Coll Cardiol 2008;52(25):2119–26.
13. Neumann PJ, Cohen JT, Weinstein MC. Updating cost-effectiveness–the curious resilience of the $50,000-per-QALY threshold. N Engl J Med 2014;371(9):796–7.
14. Pachito DV, Â Bagattini, Drager LF, et al. Economic evaluation of CPAP therapy for obstructive sleep ap-nea: a scoping review and evidence map. Sleep Breath 2021. https://doi.org/10.1007/s11325-021-02362-8.
15. Guest JF, Panca M, Sladkevicius E, et al. Clinical outcomes and cost-effectiveness of continuous pos-itive airway pressure to manage obstructive sleep apnea in patients with type 2 diabetes in the U.K. Diabetes Care 2014;37(5):1263–71.
16. McDaid C, Griffin S, Weatherly H, et al. Continuous positive airway pressure devices for the treatment of obstructive sleep apnoea-hypopnoea syndrome:

a systematic review and economic analysis. Health Technol Assess 2009;13(4):iii–iv. xi-xiv, 1-119, 143-274.

17. McMillan A, Bratton DJ, Faria R, et al. A multicentre randomised controlled trial and economic evaluation of continuous positive airway pressure for the treatment of obstructive sleep apnoea syndrome in older people: PREDICT. Health Technol Assess 2015; 19(40):1–188.

18. Chilcott J, Clayton E, Chada N, et al. Nasal continuous positive airways pressure in the management of sleep apnoea. Guidance note for purchasers. In: Research TIfHS, editor. Notthingham, and Sheffield: Universities of Leicester; 2000.

19. Guest JF, Helter MT, Morga A, et al. Cost-effectiveness of using continuous positive airway pressure in the treatment of severe obstructive sleep apnoea/hypopnoea syndrome in the UK. Thorax 2008;63(10):860–5.

20. Streatfeild J, Hillman D, Adams R, et al. Cost-effectiveness of continuous positive airway pressure therapy for obstructive sleep apnea: health care system and societal perspectives. Sleep 2019;42(12). https://doi.org/10.1093/sleep/zsz181.

21. Tousignant P, Cosio MG, Levy RD, et al. Quality adjusted life years added by treatment of obstructive sleep apnea. Sleep 1994;17(1):52–60.

22. Ayas NT, FitzGerald JM, Fleetham JA, et al. Cost-effectiveness of continuous positive airway pressure therapy for moderate to severe obstructive sleep apnea/hypopnea. Arch Intern Med 2006;166(9): 977–84.

23. Tan MC, Ayas NT, Mulgrew A, et al. Cost-effectiveness of continuous positive airway pressure therapy in patients with obstructive sleep apnea-hypopnea in British Columbia. Can Respir J 2008;15(3): 159–65.

24. Sadatsafavi M, Marra CA, Ayas NT, et al. Cost-effectiveness of oral appliances in the treatment of obstructive sleep apnoea-hypopnoea. Sleep Breath 2009;13(3):241–52.

25. Sharples L, Glover M, Clutterbuck-James A, et al. Clinical effectiveness and cost-effectiveness results from the randomised controlled Trial of Oral Mandibular Advancement Devices for Obstructive sleep apnoea-hypopnoea (TOMADO) and long-term economic analysis of oral devices and continuous positive airway pressure. Health Technol Assess 2014; 18(67):1–296.

26. Poullié AI, Cognet M, Gauthier A, et al. Cost-effectiveness of treatments for mild-to-moderate obstructive sleep apnea in France. Int J Technol Assess Health Care 2016;32(1–2):37–45.

27. de Vries GE, Hoekema A, Vermeulen KM, et al. Clinical- and cost-effectiveness of a mandibular advancement device versus continuous positive airway pressure in moderate obstructive sleep apnea. J Clin Sleep Med 2019;15(10):1477–85.

28. Aurora RN, Casey KR, Kristo D, et al. Practice parameters for the surgical modifications of the upper airway for obstructive sleep apnea in adults. Sleep 2010;33(10):1408–13.

29. Tan KB, Toh ST, Guilleminault C, et al. A cost-effectiveness analysis of surgery for middle-aged men with severe obstructive sleep apnea intolerant of CPAP. J Clin Sleep Med 2015;11(5):525–35.

30. Camacho M, Riaz M, Capasso R, et al. The effect of nasal surgery on continuous positive airway pressure device use and therapeutic treatment pressures: a systematic review and meta-analysis. Sleep 2015;38(2):279–86.

31. Kempfle JS, BuSaba NY, Dobrowski JM, et al. A cost-effectiveness analysis of nasal surgery to increase continuous positive airway pressure adherence in sleep apnea patients with nasal obstruction. Laryngoscope 2017;127(4):977–83.

32. Strollo PJ, Soose RJ, Maurer JT, et al. Upper-airway stimulation for obstructive sleep apnea. N Engl J Med 2014;370(2):139–49.

33. Certal VF, Zaghi S, Riaz M, et al. Hypoglossal nerve stimulation in the treatment of obstructive sleep apnea: a systematic review and meta-analysis. Laryngoscope 2015;125(5):1254–64.

34. Available at: https://www.cms.gov/medicare-coverage-database/view/lcd.aspx?LCDId=38385&ver=40&DocID=L38385&bc=gAAAAAgAAAAA&. Accessed October 1, 2021.

35. Pietzsch JB, Liu S, Garner AM, et al. Long-term cost-effectiveness of upper airway stimulation for the treatment of obstructive sleep apnea: a model-based projection based on the STAR trial. Sleep 2015;38(5):735–44.

36. Pietzsch JB, Richter AK, Randerath W, et al. Clinical and economic benefits of upper airway stimulation for obstructive sleep apnea in a European setting. Respiration 2019;98(1):38–47.

37. Blissett DB, Steier JS, Karagama YG, et al. Breathing synchronised hypoglossal nerve stimulation with inspire for untreated severe obstructive sleep apnoea/hypopnoea syndrome: a simulated cost-utility analysis from a national health service perspective. Pharmacoecon Open 2021;5(3): 475–89.

38. Collop N, Stierer TL, Shafazand S. SAVE me from CPAP. J Clin Sleep Med 2016;12(12):1701–4.

# Clinical Decision-making for Continuous Positive Airway Pressure Mask Selection

Jeane Lima de Andrade Xavier, PT, Mariana Delgado Fernandes, MD,
Geraldo Lorenzi-Filho, MD, Pedro R. Genta, MD*

## KEYWORDS

- Obstructive sleep apnea • CPAP • Interfaces • Mouth leak • Nasal symptoms • Breathing route

## KEY POINTS

- Assessing and treating nasal symptoms is important before starting continuous positive airway pressure treatment. The patient's perception of being a mouth breather is not indicative of an oronasal mask.
- Nasal masks are more effective to treat obstructive sleep apnea with continuous positive airway pressure. Oronasal masks are associated with higher pressure levels, lower efficacy, higher leak, and lower adherence.
- Detect and attempt to control excessive leak before switching between nasal and oronasal masks; the leak may occur through the mouth or through the mask.
- Long-term adherence to continuous positive airway pressure is highly associated with short-term initial adherence. During the initial period of treatment, it is important to monitor the patient closely.

## INTRODUCTION

Continuous positive airway pressure (CPAP) is the gold standard treatment for obstructive sleep apnea (OSA).[1,2] In the seminal study by Sullivan et al,[3] a nasal mask was used to treat OSA with CPAP. A decade later, oronasal masks were introduced as an alternative, especially for patients with nasal obstruction.[4] Since then, several new mask designs have been introduced to the market, including nasal pillows and nasal cradles. The availability of different mask designs allows the clinician to customize mask types for different patient characteristics, including facial anatomy, nasal patency, and patient preferences. Nasal masks have been associated with better CPAP adherence than oronasal masks.[5,6] In addition, nasal masks are associated with a lower residual apnea–hypopnea index, lower leak, and lower therapeutic CPAP level as compared with oronasal masks.[7] Despite the available evidence, there has been a steady increase in the prescription of oronasal masks in recent years (**Fig. 1**). The purpose of this review is to discuss the basis for the clinical decision making for CPAP mask selection.

## BREATHING ROUTE

Nasal breathing predominates both during wakefulness and sleep in normal individuals.[8] In contrast, patients with OSA predominantly breathe through the mouth, both awake and asleep.[9] Predictors for mouth breathing during sleep include, nasal obstruction, OSA severity, advanced age, higher body mass index (BMI), and larger neck circumference.[9,10] Mouth breathing may compromise airway patency owing to posterior displacement of the jaw and tongue and decreased pharyngeal dilator muscle activity.[10,11] In addition, mouth breathing can decrease upper airway

Laboratorio do Sono, Instituto do Coracao (InCor), LIM 63, Divisão de Pneumologia, Hospital das Clinicas HCFMUSP, Faculdade de Medicina, Universidade de Sao Paulo, Avenida Doutor Enéas de Carvalho Aguiar, 44 – 8th Floor, Sao Paulo, São Paulo CEP 05403-900, Brazil
* Corresponding author.
*E-mail address:* prgenta@usp.br

Sleep Med Clin 17 (2022) 569–576
https://doi.org/10.1016/j.jsmc.2022.07.011

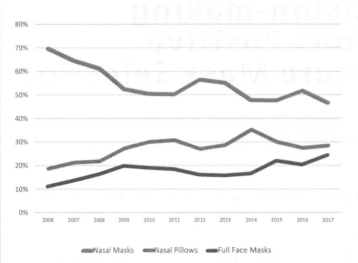

**Fig. 1.** Sales trend of different CPAP interfaces. (Source: cpap.com.)

humidification that may increase upper airway collapsibility owing to an increase in upper airway surface tension.[12,13] Oronasal breathing negatively influences CPAP adherence, especially in patients with nasal obstruction.[6,14,15] It would be intuitive to prescribe an oronasal mask for patients with mouth breathing, but determining breathing route during routine polysomnography is not trivial. Self-reported breathing route is often used as evidence to prescribe oronasal masks. However, the self-reported breathing route does not agree with the objectively detected breathing route.[8,9] Nasal masks should still be tried first for patients with objectively detected oral breathing, because nasal CPAP has been shown to significantly decrease mouth breathing in most patients over time.[16,17] Nasal CPAP may seal the airway by pushing the soft palate against the lower the tongue, preventing an oral leak.[16]

## IMPORTANCE OF EVALUATING NASAL SYMPTOMS BEFORE CONTINUOUS POSITIVE AIRWAY PRESSURE INITIATION

Nasal symptoms are common among untreated patients with OSA and are associated with decreased CPAP adherence.[17] Nasal congestion or nasal and mouth dryness can affect approximately 40% of patients who use CPAP. The clinical evaluation should include questions about nasal congestion, rhinorrhea (anterior or posterior), nasal itching, and sneezing. The causes of nasal obstruction include septum deviation, hypertrophy of the inferior turbinates, nasal valve collapse, mucosal edema, synechia, and nasal polyps (**Fig. 2**).[18,19] Nasal disorders such as a deviated septum, nasal polyps, and rhinitis decrease the nasal cross-sectional area and increase nasal

airflow resistance.[20] According to Poiseuille's law, airflow resistance is directly proportional to the length and is inversely proportional to the fourth-power of the radius of a tube.[21] Therefore, a 10% increase in the cross-sectional area of the nasal airway can result in an increase of 21% of nasal airflow.[22] The currently available treatment modalities for nasal problems range from clinical to surgical management. Nasal steroids for patients with OSA and nasal congestion has been shown to improve CPAP adherence.[23] Heated CPAP humidification for patients with nasal symptoms has also been shown to improve nasopharyngeal symptoms such as dry mouth or sore throat.[24] A meta-analysis assessing the effect of nasal surgery (septoplasty, turbinoplasty, and rhinoplasties) on CPAP level requirements showed that surgical treatment lead to a 1.9 $cmH_2O$ decrease of the pressure. An increase in nightly CPAP use of 32 minutes after nasal surgery was also observed.[25] Therefore, the assessment and treatment of nasal symptoms before CPAP initiation is imperative.

## COMPARING OUTCOMES BETWEEN NASAL AND ORONASAL MASKS

Several models of positive airway pressure device interfaces are available currently. Observational and controlled studies, as well as a meta-analyses, have compared the outcomes associated with nasal and oronasal masks.[7,24,25] In general, nasal masks have been shown to be superior to oronasal masks.[7,26–28] Three mask categories are available: nasal masks (pressure is applied to the nose and the mouth is free), nasal pillow and nasal cradles (applied directly to the nostrils), and oronasal masks (pressure is applied

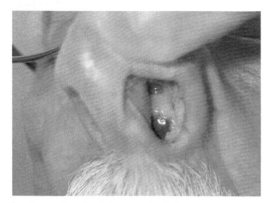

**Fig. 2.** Nasal polyp blocking the left nostril.

described.[7] Greater adherence with nasal masks was observed in nonrandomized studies, but not in randomized trials.[31] In addition, satisfaction was higher with nasal interfaces as compared with oronasal interfaces.[7,13,32,33] In studies in which patients underwent nasal CPAP titration and were then randomized to nasal versus oronasal CPAP, nasal interfaces resulted in better adherence and decreased sleepiness[10] or in a lower residual apnea–hypopnea index.[34] Several studies have found air leak to be lower with nasal interfaces.[15,30] Nasal pillows and nasal cradles are applied directly to the nostrils and are smaller in size. Nasal pillows and nasal cradles may be a better option for patients who report claustrophobia, for those with a beard or mustache, and even for those patients who wish to read using their glasses while on CPAP.[34,35] Nasal pillows were as effective as nasal masks in a randomized trial.[36,37] In summary, although oronasal masks can be effective for OSA correction, nasal masks

to both the nose and mouth)[29,30] (**Figs. 3** and **4**). Nasal masks are smaller and require less therapeutic pressure, which facilitates treatment adherence. A lower residual apnea–hypopnea index with nasal as compared with oronasal CPAP was also

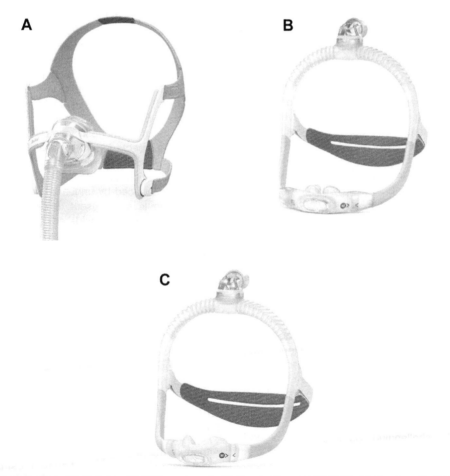

**Fig. 3.** Models of nasal interfaces. (*A*) N10 nasal mask. (*B*) Nasal pillow (AirFit P30i). (*C*) Nasal cradle (AirFit P30i) by Resmed. (© ResMed Pty Ltd. All rights reserved.)

**A**

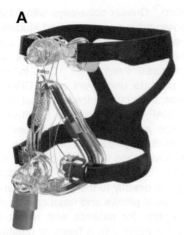

**B**

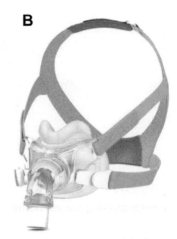

**Fig. 4.** Oronasal interface models. (*A*) Mirage Quattro face mask and (*B*) AirFit F30 is a model of Resmed is minimal contact face mask. (© ResMed Pty Ltd. All rights reserved.)

may be more advantageous and should be the first-line therapy in most cases. If CPAP titration is performed with a nasal mask, the pressure may need to be adjusted if converting to an oronasal mask.

## EXCESSIVE AIR LEAK DURING NASAL CONTINUOUS POSITIVE AIRWAY PRESSURE

CPAP masks are designed to promote intentional air leak to prevent rebreathing. Intentional leak varies according to model and CPAP level. However, unintentional leak comprises both mask and oral leak. Unintentional leak has been associated with mouth dryness, eye irritation, nasal congestion, and an increase in noise that may annoy the bed partner, and may ultimately impair CPAP adherence.[30,36] CPAP manufacturers have suggested different criteria to quantify and categorize excessive leak. Although these criteria are not validated against outcomes or symptoms, they have been used as a reference to trigger attempts for improvement. Mask leaks can occur owing to incorrect mask or model selection, incorrect mask fitting, or mask shift during a nonsupine position and in REM sleep.[38] Unintentional leak can be directly linked to several factors such as mouth opening, nasal obstruction, older age, higher BMI, a high level of CPAP, body position (other than supine, REM sleep, and a lateral position),[38–40] and advanced age, which may also be associated with facial changes owing to loss of the dental arch.[9,37,41] Distinguishing between mask or oral leak can be challenging. Some patients or bed partners may report that the major source of leak is through the mouth. Patients may wake up during mouth breathing and complain about mouth dryness. Bed partners may observe mouth opening

during periods of excessive leaks and an associated increase in noise. A study of 35 patients with moderate and severe OSA, evaluated after nasal CPAP titration and followed during the first week, described 2 different leak profiles: a continuous and a sawtooth leak profile, that may correspond with mask and oral leaks, respectively.[42] These patterns can be recognized during the graphical analysis of leak over the night taken from the CPAP device (either via telemonitoring or data card).[43] Oral leakage has been associated with increasing age, OSA severity, BMI, active smoking, and nasal obstruction.[8,11,43,44] If oral leaks are suspected during nasal CPAP, nasal symptoms need to be reviewed and treated. Heated humidification can help to decrease nasal obstruction induced by unheated nasal airflow. If oral leakage is still present, a decrease in the CPAP level may be considered. Lower levels of CPAP can decrease leakage and prevent mouth opening. Last, a chin strap can be considered in conjunction with the nasal mask. However, the effectiveness of chin straps has not been well-studied.[45–47] Switching mask models, for example, from nasal to oronasal, should be avoided. Frequent interface changes during the period of CPAP adaptation is associated with a higher risk of treatment abandonment in the first year of use.[48] **Fig. 5** summarizes a practical approach to choose between CPAP interfaces.

## ORONASAL CONTINUOUS POSITIVE AIRWAY PRESSURE FOR WHOM?

Although the available evidence indicates that nasal masks are a better option for most patients with OSA under CPAP treatment, an increasing trend of oronasal mask prescription has been

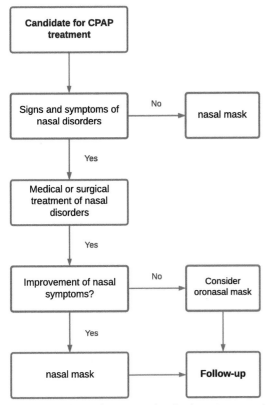

**Fig. 5.** Flowchart of CPAP mask selection. Assess and treat nasal symptoms before starting CPAP. Nasal masks are often preferred. Oronasal masks can be considered for patients with severe nasal obstruction who do not respond or cannot be treated.

noticed (see **Fig. 1**). The reasons for the increase in oronasal masks sales are not clear. Oronasal masks are often prescribed to patients reporting nasal symptoms and for those self-describing as oral breathers (**Table 1**). The clinician may prefer oronasal masks as initial choice owing to the potential risk of mouth leak during nasal CPAP. Switching masks may be cumbersome owing to additional costs for the health care service or patient. A higher profit margin for oronasal masks may lead to a bias in sales.

Most patients using oronasal masks are well-adapted. However, some patients will have a high residual apnea–hypopnea index or will require a higher than expected CPAP level while on oronasal CPAP.[29,49] Some studies have addressed this apparent paradox.[6,14,49] Oronasal masks can compromise the effectiveness of CPAP treatment owing to pressure transmitted to the oral cavity and posterior displacement of the tongue, narrowing the retroglossal area.[11,33] Among patients well-adapted to oronasal CPAP, we observed that nasal rather than oral breathing predominated.[50]

Oronasal masks could still be tried for patients that are experiencing a high oral leak on nasal CPAP despite interventions to control it, as described in **Fig. 6**. The main characteristics associated with oral breathing are severe OSA, older age, higher BMI, nasal obstruction, and a greater neck circumference.[10,17] However, patients starting oronasal CPAP should be observed carefully because oronasal masks may worsen airway obstruction.

**Table 1**
**Advantages and disadvantages of different interface types**

| Interface | Advantages | Disadvantages |
|---|---|---|
| Nasal | Smaller area of contact with the face than oronasal masks Lower therapeutic level Lower costs | Risk of mouth leak |
| Nasal pillow | Better for patients with claustrophobia Less leaking issues for patients with moustache or beard | Nasal irritation |
| Nasal cradle | More comfortable Better looking using CPAP | Upper lip skin irritation |
| Oronasal | May be an option for patients with mouth leak while on nasal CPAP | Higher mask leakage Can cause Claustrophobia May require higher therapeutic pressures Lower adherence |
| Minimal contact oronasal mask | Smaller mask More comfortable than ordinary oronasal masks | Higher cost |

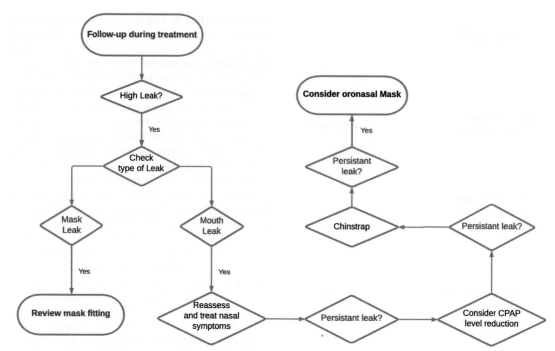

**Fig. 6.** The flowchart demonstrates the follow-up during treatment with CPAP, and the reasons for high leakage during its use, in addition to strategies that can be used to alleviate these problems during adaptation.

## FUTURE DIRECTIONS

The current diversity of masks models and sizes opens the opportunity to explore a personalized approach to select the best interface. In a randomized crossover study conducted by Goh et al[51] in Singapore, nasal, nasal pillow, and oronasal CPAP were compared. Although nasal CPAP led to better adherence, 26% of patients had greater use on oronasal CPAP. Patients showing a better adherence to oronasal CPAP had less nasal obstruction and a proportionally increased midface width and chin–lower lip distance. Future studies should consider anatomic characteristics. Three-dimensional face scanning and 3-dimensional mask printing are an interesting approach to individualize the CPAP interface according to the patient's own facial anatomy.[51,52] Future studies should also address the best approach for patients with nasal obstruction that are not candidates for surgery and those presenting a high unintentional leak under nasal CPAP.

## SUMMARY

Despite an increasing trend of sales of oronasal masks, nasal masks are usually a better option for most patients with OSA starting CPAP. Future studies should focus on personalizing CPAP interfaces according to individual patient characteristics.

## DISCLOSURE

Dr P.R. Genta was supported by CNPq (National Council of Scientific and Technological Development) (312,853/2020-3) and by FAPESP (Sao Paulo Research Foundation) (2018/20612-4).

## REFERENCES

1. Bakker JP, Neill AM, Campbell AJ. Nasal versus oronasal continuous positive airway pressure masks for obstructive sleep apnea: is this really a key point of effectiveness? Sleep Breath 2013;17(4): 1123–4.
2. Yui MS, Tominaga Q, Lopes BCP, et al. Nasal vs. oronasal mask during PAP treatment: a comparative DISE study. Sleep Breath 2020;24(3):1129–36.
3. Sullivan CE, Berthon-Jones M, Issa FG, et al. Reversal of obstructive sleep apnoea by continuous positive airway pressure applied through the nares. Lancet 1981;317(8225):862–5.
4. Sanders MH, Kern NB, Stiller RA, et al. CPAP therapy via oronasal mask for obstructive sleep apnea. Chest 1994;106(3):774–9.
5. Mehrtash M, Bakker JP, Ayas N. Predictors of continuous positive airway pressure adherence in patients with obstructive sleep apnea. Lung 2019;197(2): 115–21.
6. Borel JC, Tamisier R, Dias-Domingos S, et al. Type of mask may impact on continuous positive airway

pressure adherence in apneic patients. PLoS One 2013;8(5):e64382.

7. Andrade RGS, Viana FM, Nascimento JA, et al. Nasal vs oronasal CPAP for OSA treatment: a meta-analysis. Chest 2018;153(3):665–74.

8. Fitzpatrick MF, McLean H, Urton AM, et al. Effect of nasal or oral breathing route on upper airway resistance during sleep. Eur Respir J 2003;22(5):827–32.

9. Nascimento JA, Genta PR, Fernandes PHS, et al. Predictors of oronasal breathing among obstructive sleep apnea patients and controls. J Appl Physiol 2019;127(6):1579–85.

10. Genta PR, Kaminska M, Edwards BA, et al. The importance of mask selection on continuous positive airway pressure outcomes for obstructive sleep apnea an Official American Thoracic Society Workshop Report. Ann Am Thorac Soc 2020;17(10): 1177–85.

11. Andrade RGS, Madeiro F, Piccin VS, et al. Impact of acute changes in CPAP flow route in sleep apnea treatment. Chest 2016;150(6):1194–201.

12. Lebret M, Arnol N, Contal O, et al. Nasal obstruction and male gender contribute to the persistence of mouth opening during sleep in CPAP-treated obstructive sleep apnoea. Respirology 2015;20(7): 1123–30.

13. Hsu Y Bin, Lan MY, Huang YC, et al. Association between breathing route, oxygen desaturation, and upper airway morphology. Laryngoscope 2021;131(2): E659–64.

14. Schell AE, Soose RJ. Positive airway pressure adherence and mask interface in the setting of sinonasal symptoms. Laryngoscope 2017;127(10): 2418–22.

15. Ng JR, Aiyappan V, Mercer J, et al. Choosing an oronasal mask to deliver continuous positive airway pressure may cause more upper airway obstruction or lead to higher continuous positive airway pressure requirements than a nasal mask in some patients: a case series. J Clin Sleep Med 2016;12(9): 1227–32.

16. Ruhle KH, Nilius G. Mouth breathing in obstructive sleep apnea prior to and during nasal continuous positive airway pressure. Respiration 2008;76(1): 40–5.

17. Bachour A, Maasilta P. Mouth breathing compromises adherence to nasal continuous positive airway pressure therapy. Chest 2004;126(4):1248–54.

18. Sugiura T, Noda A, Nakata S, et al. Influence of nasal resistance on initial acceptance of continuous positive airway pressure in treatment for obstructive sleep apnea syndrome. Respiration 2006;74(1): 56–60.

19. Kryger MH, Avidan AY, Berry RB. Atlas of clinical sleep Medicine. 2nd edition. Philadelphia, PA: Elsevier/ Saunders; 2013. p. 520.

20. Coughlin K, Gillespie MB. Phenotypes of obstructive sleep apnea. Otolaryngol Clin NA 2020;53(3): 329–38.

21. Susarla SM, Thomas RJ, Abramson ZR, et al. Biomechanics of the upper airway: changing concepts in the pathogenesis of obstructive sleep apnea. Int J Oral Maxillofac Surg 2010;39(12):1149–59.

22. Powell NB, Zonato AI, Weaver EM, et al. Radiofrequency treatment of turbinate hypertrophy in subjects using continuous positive airway pressure: a randomized, double-blind, placebo-controlled clinical pilot trial. Laryngoscope 2001;111(10):1783–90.

23. Segsarnviriya C, Chumthong R, Mahakit P. Effects of intranasal steroids on continuous positive airway pressure compliance among patients with obstructive sleep apnea. Sleep Breath 2021;25(3):1293–9.

24. Soudorn C, Muntham D, Reutrakul S, et al. Effect of heated humidification on CPAP therapy adherence in subjects with obstructive sleep apnea with nasopharyngeal symptoms. Respir Care 2016;61(9): 1151–9.

25. Camacho M, Riaz M, Capasso R, et al. The effect of nasal surgery on continuous positive airway pressure device use and therapeutic treatment pressures: a systematic review and meta-analysis. Sleep 2015;38(2):279–286A.

26. Patil SP, Ayappa IA, Caples SM, et al. Treatment of adult obstructive sleep apnea with positive airway pressure: an American academy of sleep medicine systematic review, meta-analysis, and GRADE assessment. J Clin Sleep Med 2019;15(2):301–34.

27. Brenner S, Angermann C, Jany B, et al. Sleep-disordered breathing and Heart failure. A dangerous liaison. Trends Cardiovasc Med 2008;18(7):240–7.

28. Bettinzoli M, Taranto-Montemurro L, Messineo L, et al. Oronasal masks require higher levels of positive airway pressure than nasal masks to treat obstructive sleep apnea. Sleep Breath 2014;18(4): 845–9.

29. Shirlaw T, Duce B, Milosavljevic J, et al. A randomised crossover trial comparing nasal masks with oronasal masks: no differences in therapeutic pressures or residual apnea-hypopnea indices. J Sleep Res 2019;28(5):1–7.

30. Zonato AI, Rosa CFA, Oliveira L, et al. Efficacy of nasal masks versus nasal pillows masks during continuous positive airway pressure titration for patients with obstructive sleep apnea. Sleep Breath 2021;25(3):1–8.

31. Dibra MN, Berry RB, Wagner MH. Treatment of obstructive sleep apnea: choosing the best interface. Sleep Med Clin 2017;12(4):543–9.

32. Lanza A, Mariani S, Sommariva M, et al. Continuous positive airway pressure treatment with nasal pillows in obstructive sleep apnea: long-term effectiveness and adherence. Sleep Med 2018;41:94–9.

33. Madeiro F, Andrade RGS, Piccin VS, et al. Transmission of oral pressure compromises oronasal CPAP efficacy in the treatment of OSA. Chest 2019; 156(6):1187–94.

34. Richards GN, Cistulu PA, Ungar RG, et al. Mouth leak with nasal continuous positive airway pressure increases nasal airway resistance 1996;154:182–6.

35. Blanco M, Jaritos V, Ernst G, et al. Patients' preferences and the efficacy of a hybrid model of a minimal contact nasal mask in patients with sleep apnea treated with CPAP. Sleep Sci 2018;11(4):254–9.

36. Ebben MR, Oyegbile T, Pollak CP. The efficacy of three different mask styles on a PAP titration night. Sleep Med 2012;13(6):645–9.

37. Neuzeret PC, Morin L. Impact of different nasal masks on CPAP therapy for obstructive sleep apnea: a randomized comparative trial. Clin Respir J 2017;11(6):990–8.

38. Lebret M, Arnol N, Martinot J, et al. Determinants of unintentional leaks during CPAP treatment in OSA. Chest 2018;153(4):834–42.

39. Valentin A, Subramanian S, Quan SF, et al. Air leak is associated with poor adherence to autoPAP therapy. Sleep 2011;34(6):801–6.

40. Nogueira JF, Simonelli G, Giovini V, et al. Access to CPAP treatment in patients with moderate to severe sleep apnea in a Latin American City. Sleep Sci 2018;11(3):174–82.

41. Knowles SR, O'Brien DT, Zhang S, et al. Effect of addition of chin strap on PAP compliance, nightly duration of use, and other factors. J Clin Sleep Med 2014;10(4):377–83.

42. Baltzan MA, Dabrusin R, Garcia-Asensi A, et al. Leak profile inspection during nasal continuous positive airway pressure. Respir Care 2011;56(5):591–5.

43. Bachour A, Avellan-Hietanen H, Palotie T, et al. Practical aspects of interface application in CPAP treatment. Can Respir J 2019;2019:7215258.

44. Nascimento JA, De Santana Carvalho T, Moriya HT, et al. Body position may influence oronasal CPAP effectiveness to treat OSA. J Clin Sleep Med 2016; 12(3):447–8.

45. Lebret M, Jaffuel D, Suehs CM, et al. Feasibility of type 3 Polygraphy for evaluating leak determinants in CPAP- treated OSA patients. Chest 2020;158(5): 2165–71.

46. Bachour A, Hurmerinta K, Maasilta P. Mouth closing device ( chinstrap ) reduces mouth leak during nasal CPAP 2004;5:261–7.

47. Gonzalez J, Sharshar T, Hart N, et al. Air leaks during mechanical ventilation as a cause of persistent hypercapnia in neuromuscular disorders. Intensive Care Med 2003;29(4):596–602.

48. Bachour A, Vitikainen P, Maasilta P. Rates of initial acceptance of PAP masks and outcomes of mask switching. Sleep Breath 2016;20(2):733–8.

49. Rowland S, Aiyappan V, Hennessy C, et al. Comparing the efficacy , mask leak , patient Adherence , and patient preference of three different CPAP interfaces to treat moderate-severe obstructive sleep apnea. J Clin Sleep Med 2018;14(1): 101–8.

50. Xavier JL de A, Madeiro Leite Viana Weaver F, Pinheiro GL, et al. Patients with OSA on oronasal CPAP breathe predominantly through the nose during natural sleep. Am J Respir Crit Care Med 2021;(1):1–4.

51. GOH K, Soh RY, Leow LC, et al. Choosing the right mask for your Asian patient with sleep apnoea : a randomized , crossover trial of CPAP interfaces. Respirology 2018;2018:278–85.

52. Ma Z, Drinnan M, Hyde P, et al. Mask interface for continuous positive airway pressure therapy: selection and design considerations. Expert Rev Med Devices 2018;15(10):725–33.

# Use of Positive Airway Pressure in the Treatment of Hypoventilation

Annie C. Lajoie, MD[a], Marta Kaminska, MD, MSc[a,b],*

## KEYWORDS

- Hypoventilation • Sleep-disordered breathing • Neuromuscular disease • COPD
- Obesity-hypoventilation syndrome • Obstructive sleep apnea • Positive airway pressure
- Noninvasive ventilation (NIV)

## KEY POINTS

- Sleep-related hypoventilation is a precursor to chronic hypercapnic respiratory failure in many conditions including obesity hypoventilation syndrome, COPD, neuromuscular, and chest wall disorders.
- Treatment of sleep-related hypoventilation usually requires home noninvasive ventilation, typically using bilevel positive airway pressure.
- Continuous positive airway pressure can improve patient outcomes when obstructive sleep apnea is the main cause of nocturnal hypoventilation.

## INTRODUCTION

Sleep-related hypoventilation encompasses a variety of conditions where reduced ventilation during sleep leads to elevated arterial partial pressure of carbon dioxide ($Paco_2$) at night.[1] The American Academy of Sleep Medicine defines sleep-related hypoventilation as an increase in $Paco_2$ greater than 55 mm Hg lasting more than 10 minutes or an increase in $Paco_2$ greater than 10 mm Hg (compared with an awake supine value), reaching a value greater than 50 mm Hg and lasting longer than 10 minutes.[2] $Paco_2$ is usually measured during sleep with noninvasive methods such as transcutaneous or end-tidal $Paco_2$ monitoring.[2] Arterial oxygen ($O_2$) desaturations often accompany episodes of hypoventilation but are not always present or required for the diagnosis.[1]

Hypoventilation results from alterations in the control of breathing (will not breathe) or abnormalities in respiratory mechanics (cannot breathe). The former originates from impairment of the brain stem respiratory control center, including anatomic, metabolic, endocrine, or pharmacologic disturbances, whereas the latter results from conditions that affect the neuromuscular, chest wall, or pulmonary function.

In chronic conditions, before becoming apparent during the daytime, hypoventilation typically first becomes manifest at night.[3] The third edition of the International Classification of Sleep Disorders identifies 6 subtypes of sleep-related hypoventilation disorders (**Box 1**).[1] Of these, the obesity-hypoventilation syndrome (OHS) and hypoventilation related to medical disorders or due to a medication or substance are the most prevalent.[3] Medical disorders that may lead to

[a] Respiratory Epidemiology and Clinical Research Unit, Research Institute of the McGill University Health Centre - Montreal, 5252 Boulevard de Maisonneuve Ouest, Montréal, Quebec H4A 3S9, Canada; [b] Respiratory Division & Sleep Laboratory, McGill University Health Centre - Montreal, 1001 Decarie Boulevard, Montreal, Quebec H4A 3J1, Canada
* Corresponding author. Respiratory Epidemiology and Clinical Research Unit, Research Institute of the McGill University Health Centre - Montreal, 5252 Boulevard de Maisonneuve Ouest, Montréal, Quebec H4A 3S9, Canada.
E-mail address: marta.kaminska@mcgill.ca

Sleep Med Clin 17 (2022) 577–586
https://doi.org/10.1016/j.jsmc.2022.07.004
1556-407X/22/© 2022 Elsevier Inc. All rights reserved.

Box 1
Sleep-related hypoventilation disorder according to the International Classification of Sleep Disorders, third edition

- Obesity hypoventilation syndrome
- Congenital central alveolar hypoventilation syndrome
- Late-onset central hypoventilation with hypothalamic dysfunction
- Idiopathic central alveolar hypoventilation
- Sleep-related hypoventilation due to a medication or substance (eg, long-acting opioids, anesthetics, sedatives, and muscle relaxants)
- Sleep-related hypoventilation due to a medical disorder (lung parenchymal, airway or vascular disease, neurologic or neuromuscular disease, chest wall disorder)

sleep-related hypoventilation include neuromuscular or neurologic diseases, thoracic cage disorders, hypothyroidism, or disorders of the pulmonary airways, parenchyma, or vasculature.[1] Congenital central hypoventilation syndrome and rapid-onset obesity with hypothalamic dysfunction, hypoventilation, and autonomic dysregulation are much rarer and will often present at birth or become manifest in early childhood.[3] However, they can seldom become apparent in older individuals, often after a triggering event such as acute illness or general anesthesia, then termed "late-onset."[1] Finally, when no underlying disease is identified, the term idiopathic sleep-related hypoventilation is used.

Sleep-related hypoventilation usually requires noninvasive ventilation (NIV) therapy in sleep to increase carbon dioxide ($CO_2$) elimination. However, in circumstances where obstructive sleep apnea (OSA) is the main cause of hypoventilation, continuous positive airway pressure (CPAP) can be an effective therapeutic option. In this article, we will review the pathophysiology of sleep-related hypoventilation, discuss the use of CPAP and NIV and review NIV modes and settings.

## Pathophysiology of Hypoventilation During Sleep

Ventilation is physiologically reduced during sleep due to changes in the central control of breathing, respiratory and upper airway muscle function, and lung mechanics.[4] At sleep onset, the wakefulness drive to breathe disappears, cortical and respiratory motor neuron outputs are reduced, and the chemoreceptors' response to changes in arterial

$O_2$ and $CO_2$ are blunted.[5] Lung volumes, especially functional residual capacity, decrease during sleep due to cephalad displacement of the diaphragm, and muscle hypotonia/atonia, with reduction in lung compliance and increased upper airway resistance.[6] Altogether, these physiologic changes occurring during sleep reduce minute ventilation by 15% to 20%.[7] This is rather uneventful in healthy individuals but becomes significant in patients with diseases that further affect respiratory mechanics and ventilation, such as chronic obstructive or restrictive lung diseases, chest wall disorders, neuromuscular diseases, and obesity.[8]

Respiratory control differs according to sleep stages. During nonrapid eye movement (NREM) sleep, respiratory amplitude and rate are relatively stable, and the control of ventilation relies primarily on the integrity of peripheral and central chemoreceptors.[4] Conversely, respiration during REM sleep is characterized by variations in tidal volumes and breathing rate,[4] and markedly reduced activity of respiratory muscles, except the diaphragm.[9] As a result, breathing becomes diaphragm-dependent, and accessory muscles of respiration, potentially heavily relied on in conditions such as severe chronic obstructive pulmonary disease (COPD) and certain neuromuscular disorders, cannot contribute during REM sleep. Upper airway obstruction also tends to be greater in REM sleep. As a result, REM sleep constitutes a challenge for respiration and often presents the first manifestations of hypoventilation before NREM sleep is also affected.[4] Hypoventilation in sleep eventually leads to hypercapnia in wakefulness. This results from compensation of the nocturnal respiratory acidosis by the kidneys, with reabsorption of bicarbonate in the proximal tubule.[10] The resulting increase in serum and cerebrospinal fluid bicarbonate (metabolic alkalosis) participates in desensitization of the hypercapnic ventilatory response and ensuing chronic hypoventilation.[11] Hence, chronic hypercapnic respiratory failure can usually be corrected by treatment of sleep-disordered breathing alone, except in cases of extremely impaired neuromuscular or pulmonary function or central control of breathing.

Hypoventilation is usually not predominant in patients with OSA.[12,13] However, varying degrees of hypercapnia can occur following obstructive events that in some patients can progress to sustained hypercapnia and chronic hypoventilation, especially when another condition affects ventilation.[12,14,15] Individuals with OSA who have hypercapnia exhibit a blunted ventilatory response to a given change in $CO_2$. The ability to unload $CO_2$ after an obstructive event depends not only on the individuals' ventilatory response to changes in $CO_2$ but also on characteristics of the obstructive events itself.[12,16] Shorter periods between apneas (the interapnea period) in relation with the duration of the apnea (shorter interapnea:apnea ratio) foster hypoventilation.[12,16] $CO_2$ retention is amplified during REM sleep where obstructive events tend to be longer, and in patients with impaired respiratory function such as those suffering from neuromuscular or chest wall diseases, obstructive lung disease, or obesity.[12]

### Treatment Modalities

In patients with chronic sleep-related hypoventilation, ventilatory support is usually provided using NIV, often by means of bilevel positive airway pressure (BPAP).[17] Unlike CPAP, which fundamentally delivers the same level of pressure throughout the respiratory cycle, BPAP provides inspiratory pressure support (PS) to a prespecified inspiratory pressure level (IPAP) in addition to a baseline (expiratory) level of pressure [expiratory positive airway pressure (EPAP)].[17] NIV can also be delivered by mask or mouthpiece in volumetric mode. When OSA is the main cause of hypercapnia, CPAP can be a viable therapeutic option because it will reduce $Paco_2$ by preventing upper airway collapse, normalizing ventilation, and reducing work of breathing.

### Obesity-Hypoventilation Syndrome

OHS is defined by the presence of daytime hypercapnia ($Paco_2 > 45$ mm Hg) in an obese individual (body mass index $>30$ kg/m$^2$) in the absence of another cause of hypoventilation.[1] Sleep-disordered breathing is a prominent feature. The pathophysiology of OHS is multifactorial and results from the adverse effects of obesity on lung mechanics, upper airway and respiratory muscles, as well as impaired central ventilatory drive.[15] Excessive adiposity of the chest wall increases work of breathing and decreases lung volumes, especially functional residual capacity and expiratory reserve volume, which reduces diaphragm mobility.[18] There is decreased respiratory system compliance, increased lower airway resistance, premature airway closure with gas trapping and inhomogeneity of ventilation.[19] Atelectasis can also result in mismatched ventilation and perfusion, and hypoxemia.[20] Compared with obese individuals without OHS, patients with OHS exhibit impairments in the central ventilatory drive.[21] This is thought to result from desensitization of the hypercapnic ventilatory response and, in part, from leptin resistance.[22] Leptin, a hormone produced by adipose cells and involved in the regulation of

hunger, is a potent ventilatory stimulant.[22] High levels of leptin, or leptin resistance, in obese individuals predicts the development of hypercapnia and OHS.[22]

The presence of adipose tissue around the upper airway, reduced lung volumes and rostral redistribution of lower extremity edema to the upper airway when recumbent (also called fluid shift), reduce pharyngeal lumen size and increase upper airway collapsibility, predisposing to obstructive breathing events during sleep.[23] Ninety percent of patients with OHS have concomitant OSA, defined as an apnea-hypopnea index (AHI) greater than 5 events per hour, and up to 70% with severe disease (AHI $>30$ events/h).[13] The presence of severe OSA constitutes a distinct phenotype of OHS: compared with the hypoventilation phenotype without OSA, these patients are often younger men who are more severely obese and suffer from significant impairment in gas exchange and respiratory muscle function despite having a lower prevalence of cardiovascular comorbidities.[13,24,25]

The most recent guideline from the American Thoracic Society recommends CPAP in OHS patients who have evidence of severe OSA.[26] This recommendation is mostly based on findings from the Pickwick study.[13] In this randomized controlled trial, patients with OHS and severe OSA were randomized to receive NIV, CPAP, or lifestyle modifications (dietary restrictions and sleep hygiene and habits modifications).[13] Nocturnal and diurnal gas exchanges ($Paco_2$ and $Pao_2$) as well as sleep quality improved on CPAP and NIV compared with lifestyle modifications alone. NIV yielded a greater reduction in $Paco_2$ at 2 months and showed improvement in lung function and exercise capacity (6-minutes walking test) compared with CPAP in the short term but between-group differences disappeared in long-term follow-up.[27] Other studies also found that, in patients with OHS and severe OSA, CPAP led to improvement in gas exchange, sleepiness, and sleep quality similar to NIV.[28,29] Furthermore, long-term data from the Pickwick trial found no difference between CPAP and NIV in terms of healthcare utilization, incidence of cardiovascular disease, or mortality rate after a median follow-up of 5.44 years in OHS patients with severe OSA.[27] A recent systematic review and meta-analysis also found a greater cost–benefit to CPAP.[30] However, CPAP failure rate and need to convert to NIV has been reported at 20% to 40%.[30–32] Risk factors for CPAP failure are advanced age, more significant impairment in lung function, and greater degree of hypercapnia and/or hypoxemia.[30]

NIV remains the first-line therapy for OHS in patients *without* severe OSA.[26] Randomized controlled trials and case series in OHS patients without severe OSA indicate that NIV effectively improves gas exchange, sleepiness, and health-related quality of life but adherence tends to be lower in this group.[25,28,33,34]

NIV is also recommended for home use on leaving the hospital in cases of acute-on-chronic hypercapnic respiratory failure, where it improves gas exchanges, lung function, and reduces mortality.[35,36] Of patients on NIV, many can be switched to CPAP but close monitoring is required due to a significant failure rate.[31,32] In patients with or without severe OSA, derived benefits of CPAP and NIV depend on treatment adherence.[25,26] Both CPAP and NIV seem to be well tolerated in this population.[26]

### Chronic Obstructive Pulmonary Disease

Sleep can be a challenging state for patients with severe COPD because their capacity to compensate for the physiologic changes in breathing is compromised.[37] This is especially true during REM sleep, where variations in tidal volume and respiratory rate can worsen hyperinflation and create intrinsic positive end expiratory pressure (PEEP).[37] The diaphragmatic dysfunction occurring in patients with COPD, which results from hyperinflation that places the diaphragm in a disadvantageous position or from COPD-related or steroid-related skeletal myopathy, is a major contributor to hypoventilation during REM sleep.[38]

Sleep-related hypoxemia and hypercapnia are frequent in COPD and contribute to adverse consequences such as pulmonary hypertension and cor pulmonale.[39] COPD patients with low baseline pulse $O_2$ saturation ($SpO_2$) are especially prone to $O_2$ desaturation in sleep because they find themselves on the steepest part of the oxyhemoglobin dissociation curve where any given change in $PaO_2$ will result in a greater decline in $SpO_2$.[40] $O_2$ desaturations during sleep in COPD can stem from hypoventilation, ventilation-perfusion mismatches, or coexisting OSA.[37]

The overlap syndrome refers to the co-occurrence of COPD and OSA, both of which are highly prevalent conditions.[14] Some features of COPD theoretically predispose to the development of OSA.[14] The integrity of upper airway neuromuscular responses may be affected by inflammation due to cigarette smoking or skeletal myopathy related to COPD, deconditioning, or corticosteroid use.[41] In patients who have cor pulmonale and lower leg edema, rostral fluid shift at night contributes to reduction in upper airway caliber and increases collapsibility of the upper airway.[23] Conversely, some characteristics of severe COPD make OSA less likely, including lower BMI, reduction in the amount of REM sleep, and hyperinflation, which creates traction on the upper airway making it less collapsible.[14,42]

Patients with overlap syndrome have more profound nocturnal desaturations and hypercapnia, especially during REM sleep, and reduced sleep quality compared with patients with OSA or COPD alone.[43] In patients with COPD, the presence of OSA exacerbates airway inflammation and contributes to oxidative stress and lung damage, which increases the risk of acute COPD exacerbations.[44,45] These patients will often exhibit significant daytime hypoxemia and pulmonary hypertension despite having mild-to-moderate COPD.[46] The overlap syndrome is associated with worse quality of life, higher risk of all-cause and cardiovascular mortality, as well as time to hospitalization due to COPD, compared with COPD alone.[46,47]

In severe COPD, CPAP improves gas exchanges, pulmonary function and lung volumes, and decreases work of breathing.[48] In addition to alleviating upper airway obstructions, PEEP can counteract intrinsic PEEP and reduce upper and lower airway resistance.[49] In overlap syndrome, although no randomized controlled trials have compared CPAP with standard care, cohort studies suggest that CPAP improves morbidity and mortality.[46,50,51] Interestingly, looking at subgroups of patients with overlap syndrome based on presence or absence of hypercapnia, only hypercapnic patients had reduced mortality with CPAP.[52] Adherence to CPAP is an important element for improved survival in overlap syndrome.[53,54]

In the absence of overlap syndrome, COPD patients who have chronic stable hypercapnia may be candidates for long-term home NIV.[53–55] Although the benefits of NIV for the management of acute hypercapnic respiratory failure in COPD are clear, evidence for NIV use in chronic stable COPD has been inconsistent. A 2009 multicentric RCT suggested that NIV added to long-term $O_2$ therapy (LTOT) improves survival but at the expense of reduced health-related quality of life, in severe COPD patients with chronic hypercapnic respiratory failure.[56] However, a 2014 systematic review and individual patient data meta-analysis concluded that NIV added no benefit in terms of blood gases, 6-minute walking distance, health-related quality of life, lung function, respiratory muscle function, and sleep efficiency, compared with usual treatment in patients with severe COPD.[57] However, the included studies had varying $PaCO_2$ inclusion thresholds (43–56 mm Hg), used relatively low levels of ventilatory support

(IPAP 10–16 cmH2O) and were not aiming to reduce or normalize $Paco_2$. Since then, studies using a "high-intensity" NIV strategy, which targets $Paco_2$ normalization using high inspiratory pressures (IPAP $\geq$ 18 cmH2O) with or without a relatively high backup rate, have emerged. This strategy benefited gas exchange and respiratory muscle function.[58–60] In the Köhnlein study, patients with severe COPD with stable chronic hypercapnia ($Paco_2 \geq$ 51.9 mm Hg and pH > 7.35) were randomized to receive NIV or usual care.[60] With their ventilation strategy, they aimed at significantly reducing (>20% reduction) or normalizing $Paco_2$ (values < 48 mm Hg). After 1 year, mortality was substantially lower in the NIV and LTOT group compared with standard COPD treatment.

Another key aspect is timing of NIV initiation. In a 2014 RCT, NIV was initiated during hospitalization for acute hypercapnic respiratory failure in patients with COPD and persistent hypercapnia greater than 48 hours after end of acute NIV use.[61] The study failed to show improvements in time to readmission or mortality after 1 year of NIV compared with standard treatment. Interestingly, $Paco_2$ also improved significantly in the control group, suggesting that $Paco_2$ improves gradually after an episode of acute COPD exacerbation and that patients without more persistent hypercapnia are less likely to benefit from home NIV. In the HOT-HMV trial, COPD patients with hypercapnia ($Paco_2$ > 53 mm Hg) persisting 2 to 4 weeks after acute hypercapnic respiratory failure were randomized to NIV and LTOT or LTOT alone.[62] Addition of home NIV to LTOT delayed time to readmission for COPD exacerbation.

Home NIV, especially high-intensity NIV, seems to be well tolerated and only minimal adverse events, such as local skin reactions, have been reported.[60,63] These observations recently prompted the European Respiratory Society and the American and Canadian Thoracic Societies to issue guidelines suggesting home NIV use in selected COPD patients with chronic stable or persistent hypercapnia 2 to 4 weeks following a hospitalization for acute COPD exacerbation.[53–55] All societies emphasize that evidence is weak and many unknowns remain, for example, regarding obese patients or those with overlap syndrome, largely excluded from the trials discussed above. The American Thoracic Society recommends screening for OSA before NIV initiation.[54] Although the suggested modalities of NIV initiation vary between guidelines and the $Paco_2$ threshold for the treatment initiation remains unclear, all societies agree that the treatment should aim at normalizing $Paco_2$ by using a high-intensity NIV strategy. NIV in this context seems to be cost-effective.[64]

## Neuromuscular and Chest Wall Diseases

Home mechanical ventilation has greatly improved the outcomes of patients with neuromuscular, neurodegenerative, and chest wall disease who develop chronic respiratory failure.[65–67] In rapidly progressing neuromuscular diseases such as amyotrophic lateral sclerosis (ALS), where death occurs in 50% of patients within 3 year of symptom onset,[68] home NIV improves some aspects of quality of life; slows the decline of pulmonary function; improves sleep architecture, gas exchange, sleep-disordered breathing, and its related symptoms; and prolongs survival.[69,70] Benefits are greater for patients without bulbar involvement.[71] Bulbar involvement may predispose patients with ALS to OSA.[72] However, sleep disordered breathing in ALS consists mainly of hypoventilation or mixed and central apneas rather than obstructive apneas.[72] ALS differs from other neuromuscular diseases due to the rapidity of progression leading to death. Therefore, early NIV initiation has been advocated, classically based on the presence of orthopnea, Forced vital capacity (FVC) less than 50% of predicted, sniff nasal inspiratory pressure > −40cmH2O or maximum inspiratory pressure (MIP) > −60 cmH2O.[69] However, even earlier initiation, for example, in patients with forced vital capacity greater than 65%, seems to improve survival[67] and has been advocated in more recent guidelines.[70,71]

For other neuromuscular or chest wall diseases, such as Duchenne muscular dystrophy, myotonic dystrophy, or kyphoscoliosis, the timing of screening for hypoventilation varies according to the underlying neuromuscular disease (usually when forced vital capacity is less than 40%–50% or significant respiratory muscle weakness is found).[70] In addition to overt daytime hypercapnia, criteria for NIV initiation include the presence of symptoms of sleep disordered breathing or hypoventilation with abnormal sleep study results, or significantly reduced pulmonary function (FVC <50%, MIP < −60cmH2O).[70] This is particularly true in the setting of disorders with progressive deterioration such as Duchenne muscular dystrophy. Treatment with and adherence to NIV may improve the quality of life, morbidity, and mortality in patients with neuromuscular and chest wall disease.[66,73] NIV can be provided up to 24 hours per day by mask or mouthpiece ventilation.[70] Tracheostomy, associated with increased complications, is rarely necessary and is often reserved for exceptional cases, such as severe bulbar symptoms.[73–75] In cases where OSA and obesity are prominent with only a mild and stable restrictive pulmonary syndrome, and in the absence of

**Table 1**
**Positive airway pressure modes and settings**

| Disorder | PAP Modes | NIV Settings |
|---|---|---|
| OHS1,28 | Severe OSA → CPAP<br>No OSA or mild/moderate OSA →<br>• BPAP-S (adequate ventilatory drive)<br>• BPAP-ST or VAPS (inadequate ventilatory drive; back-up rate needed)<br>* Patients hospitalized for hypercapnic respiratory failure should be started on NIV and reassessed within 3 mo with a sleep study/PAP titration | • Target Vt ~ 8 mL/kg ideal body weight<br>• High IPAP; if VAPS, high IPAP min and max<br>• EPAP: high if severe OSA. Adjust to eliminate obstructive events [automatic EPAP (AE) mode could be used]<br>• Restrictive physiology, aim for:<br>  ○ Slower rise time or adjust for comfort<br>  ○ Prolonged Ti<br>  ○ Medium to lower trigger sensitivity<br>  ○ Lower cycle sensitivity |
| Severe COPD 60–62 | Overlap syndrome → CPAP<br>Chronic stable hypercapnic respiratory failure without OSA → BPAP-S, BPAP-ST or VAPS<br>Supplemental $O_2$ if necessary | • Target Vt ~ 8 mL/kg ideal body weight<br>• High IPAP (>18cmH2O) for "high-intensity" NIV strategy. Aim to normalize or significantly lower $Pa_{CO_2}$<br>• EPAP to eliminate obstructive events (if present) or mitigate intrinsic PEEP<br>• Autoadjusting EPAP with EFL-targeting protocol could be used<br>• Obstructive physiology, aim for longer exhalation time<br>  ○ Faster rise time<br>  ○ Shorter Ti<br>  ○ Higher cycle sensitivity |
| Neuromuscular diseases73,77,81 | Isolated OSA with no significant restrictive syndrome → CPAP<br>Hypoventilation: BPAP-ST, BPAP-PC, or VAPS | • Target Vt ~ 8 mL/kg ideal body weight<br>• IPAP as tolerated to reach targeted Vt<br>• Low EPAP<br>• Weak respiratory muscles<br>  ○ Higher trigger sensitivity<br>  ○ Slow rise time or adjust for comfort<br>  ○ Longer Ti<br>  ○ Low cycle sensitivity |

*Abbreviations:* BPAP, bi-level positive airway pressure; CPAP, continuous positive airway pressure; EFL, expiratory flow limitation; EPAP, expiratory positive airway pressure; IPAP, inspiratory positive airway pressure; NIV, noninvasive ventilation; OHS, obesity hypoventilation syndrome; OSA; obstructive sleep apnea; PEEP, positive end-expiratory pressure; S-, spontaneous; ST-spontaneous-timed; Ti, inspiratory time; VAPS, volume assured pressure support; Vt, tidal volume.

chronic hypoventilation, CPAP treatment of OSA can be considered, with appropriate monitoring.[65] OSA and use of PAP in neurologic populations is further discussed in a separate article in this issue.

## Noninvasive Ventilation Modes and Settings

Most frequently, home NIV is achieved using BPAP, although volumetric ventilation can also be provided by noninvasive interface. Pressure-targeted NIV (BPAP) seems to be better tolerated.[76] BPAP delivers distinct levels of IPAP and EPAP. The difference between IPAP and EPAP is called the PS and is an important determinant of tidal volume and, ultimately, minute ventilation. EPAP is set to eliminate upper airway obstruction. Algorithms exist that allow certain BPAP devices to automatically adjust EPAP to maintain upper airway patency throughout the night (auto-EPAP or AE). In patients with severe COPD, expiratory flow limitation (EFL) may lead to increased end-expiratory lung volume and intrinsic PEEP.[77] Some devices use a forced oscillation technique to determine the amount of EFL and automatically adjust the EPAP to abolish EFL.[78]

When using pressure ventilation (BPAP), the inspiratory pressure is preset and variable volumes will be delivered according to the respiratory system compliance and impedance. Most commonly used BPAP modes include the timed (T), spontaneous (S), spontaneous-timed (ST), and pressure-controlled (PC) modes (**Table 1**). Differences lie in their triggering and cycling. Triggering of breaths by the patient (S, ST, PC) can be flow-based or pressure-based, with adjustable sensitivity. Higher sensitivity allows easier triggering, which is useful in patients with neuromuscular diseases or auto-PEEP. A lower trigger sensitivity can improve patient–device synchrony by limiting excessive triggering. In T mode, the patient is not allowed to trigger breaths. In ST and PC modes, breaths will be machine-initiated if the patient's spontaneous respiratory rate drops less than the set back-up rate. Cycling refers to the transition from IPAP to EPAP (end of inspiration to beginning of expiration) and can be a function of flow or time. When the breath is flow-cycled (S, ST patient-triggered breaths), the device will terminate inspiration based on flow drop-off, expressed as a percentage of the peak inspiratory flow. When the breath is time-cycled (T, PC, ST device-triggered breaths), inspiration ceases after the preset Ti is reached. When an inspiratory window is determined by Ti minimum and Ti maximum (S, ST on some devices), the breath can be flow-cycled within this window. In obstructive lung diseases, ventilators are prone to delayed cycling to EPAP.[79] A shorter Ti or Timax may reduce the resulting asynchrony and promote longer expiration time to limit hyperinflation. Conversely, in restrictive disorders, ventilators tend to cycle to EPAP prematurely.[79] Therefore, setting a higher Ti or Timin helps ensure good lung expansion and reduces work of breathing.

The time to reach maximal IPAP from EPAP is called rise time. A faster rise time helps increase inspiratory flow and tidal volume and can be useful when there is high respiratory drive, muscle weakness, high resistance, or when longer expiratory time is needed (eg, COPD). Slower rise time can be helpful in restrictive physiology or for patient comfort.

In volume-targeted or ventilation-targeted BPAP modes (see **Table 1**), the target tidal volume or alveolar ventilation is set, together with a range of PS (or IPAP). The device will then adjust inspiratory PS within the allowed range throughout the night to meet the target. Depending on the device and algorithm, the ventilation targets can be based on expiratory tidal volume (average volume assured PS) or alveolar ventilation (based on anatomic dead space calculated from patient height and targeted backup rate; intelligent volume assured pressure). There is currently no evidence that these ventilation strategies substantially improve patient's outcomes compared with fixed pressure BPAP.[80,81]

## SUMMARY

NIV has greatly improved outcomes of patients with chronic hypercapnic respiratory failure. However, situations where CPAP could be used should be identified because this may lead to significant clinical improvement, at a lower cost. Nevertheless, treatment with PAP should not only be tailored to the underlying pathophysiology and targeted to overcome hypoventilation but also to optimize comfort and adherence to PAP therapy.

## CLINICS CARE POINTS

- Hypoventilation results from alterations in the control of breathing or in respiratory mechanics.

- Hypoventilation typically first manifests at night, especially during rapid eye movement (REM) sleep, before extending to the daytime period.

- Non-invasive ventilation is usually required to treat sleep-related hypoventilation but continuous positive airway pressure may be sufficient in certain contexts (e.g. severe OSA with obesity-hypoventilation syndrome or COPD).

- Non-invasive ventilation parameters should be tailored to the underlying pathophysiology of hypoventilation and the patient characteristics.

## DISCLOSURE

A.C. Lajoie has nothing to disclose regarding the present article. M. Kaminska reports being on the Advisory Board for Biron Soins du Sommeil, unrestricted research support from Philips, VitalAire, and Fisher Paykel.

## REFERENCES

1. American Academy of Sleep Medicine. International Classification of Sleep Disorders. 3rd ed. Darien, IL: American Academy of Sleep Medicine; 2014.

2. Berry RB BR, Gamaldo CE, Harding SM, Lloyd RM, Marcus CL, Vaughn BV. for the American Academy of Sleep Medicine. The AASM Manual for the Scoring of Sleep and Associated Events: Rules, Terminology and Technical Specifications, Version 2.3. Darien, IL: American Academy of Sleep Medicine; 2014.

3. Böing S, Randerath WJ. Chronic hypoventilation syndromes and sleep-related hypoventilation. J Thorac Dis 2015;7(8):1273–85.

4. Douglas NJ, White DP, Pickett CK, et al. Respiration during sleep in normal man. Thorax 1982;37(11): 840–4.

5. Dempsey JA, Skatrud JB. A sleep-induced apneic threshold and its consequences. Am Rev Respir Dis 1986;133(6):1163–70.

6. Ballard RD, Irvin CG, Martin RJ, et al. Influence of sleep on lung volume in asthmatic patients and normal subjects. J Appl Physiol 1990;68(5):2034–41.

7. Krieger J, Maglasiu N, Sforza E, et al. Breathing during sleep in normal middle-aged subjects. Sleep 1990;13(2):143–54.

8. Skatrud JB, Dempsey JA, Badr S, et al. Effect of airway impedance on CO2 retention and respiratory muscle activity during NREM sleep. J Appl Physiol 1988;65(4):1676–85.

9. Brooks PL, Peever JH. Identification of the transmitter and receptor mechanisms responsible for REM sleep paralysis. J Neurosci 2012;32(29):9785–95.

10. Krapf R. Mechanisms of adaptation to chronic respiratory acidosis in the rabbit proximal tubule. J Clin Invest 1989;83(3):890–6.

11. Burgraff NJ, Neumueller SE, Buchholz K, et al. Ventilatory and integrated physiological responses to chronic hypercapnia in goats. J Physiol 2018; 596(22):5343–63.

12. Ayappa I, Berger KI, Norman RG, et al. Hypercapnia and ventilatory periodicity in obstructive sleep apnea syndrome. AJRCCM 2002;166(8):1112–5.

13. Masa JF, Corral J, Alonso ML, et al. Efficacy of different treatment Alternatives for obesity hypoventilation syndrome. Pickwick study. AJRCCM 2015; 192(1):86–95.

14. McNicholas WT. COPD-OSA overlap syndrome: Evolving evidence regarding Epidemiology, clinical consequences, and management. Chest 2017; 152(6):1318–26.

15. Masa JF, Pépin J-L, Borel J-C, et al. Obesity hypoventilation syndrome. Eur Respir Rev 2019;28(151).

16. Berger KI, Ayappa I, Sorkin IB, et al. Postevent ventilation as a function of CO(2) load during respiratory events in obstructive sleep apnea. J Appl Physiol 2002;93(3):917–24.

17. Selim BJ, Wolfe L, Coleman JM 3rd, et al. Initiation of noninvasive ventilation for sleep related hypoventilation disorders: advanced modes and devices. Chest 2018;153(1):251–65.

18. Sant'Anna M de J, Carvalhal RF, Oliveira FDFB, et al. Respiratory mechanics of patients with morbid obesity. Jornal brasileiro de pneumologia 2019; 45(5):e20180311.

19. Holley HS, Milic-Emili J, Becklake MR, et al. Regional distribution of pulmonary ventilation and perfusion in obesity. J Clin Invest 1967;46(4):475–81.

20. Zavorsky GS, Hoffman SL. Pulmonary gas exchange in the morbidly obese. Obes Rev 2008; 9(4):326–39.

21. Balmain BN, Halverson QM, Tomlinson AR, et al. Obesity Blunts the ventilatory response to exercise in men and Women. Ann Am Thorac Soc 2021; 18(7):1167–74.

22. Phipps PR, Starritt E, Caterson I, et al. Association of serum leptin with hypoventilation in human obesity. Thorax 2002;57(1):75–6.

23. White LH, Bradley TD. Role of nocturnal rostral fluid shift in the pathogenesis of obstructive and central sleep apnoea. J Physiol 2013;591(5):1179–93.

24. de Llano LP, Castro-Añón O, Castro-Cabana L, et al. Long-term effectiveness of CPAP in patients with severe obesity-hypoventilation syndrome. Sleep & breathing 2021;25(2):947–50.

25. Masa JF, Corral J, Caballero C, et al. Non-invasive ventilation in obesity hypoventilation syndrome without severe obstructive sleep apnoea. Thorax 2016;71(10):899–906.

26. Mokhlesi B, Masa JF, Brozek JL, et al. Evaluation and management of obesity hypoventilation syndrome. An Official American thoracic society clinical practice guideline. AJRCCM 2019;200(3): e6–24.

27. Masa JF, Mokhlesi B, Benítez I, et al. Long-term clinical effectiveness of continuous positive airway pressure therapy versus non-invasive ventilation therapy in patients with obesity hypoventilation syndrome: a multicentre, open-label, randomised controlled trial. Lancet 2019;393(10182):1721–32.

28. Piper AJ, Wang D, Yee BJ, et al. Randomised trial of CPAP vs bilevel support in the treatment of obesity hypoventilation syndrome without severe nocturnal desaturation. Thorax 2008;63(5):395–401.

29. Howard ME, Piper AJ, Stevens B, et al. A randomised controlled trial of CPAP versus non-invasive ventilation for initial treatment of obesity hypoventilation syndrome. Thorax 2017;72(5):437–44.

30. Soghier I, Brożek JL, Afshar M, et al. Noninvasive ventilation versus CPAP as initial treatment of obesity hypoventilation syndrome. Ann Am Thorac Soc 2019;16(10):1295–303.

31. Arellano-Maric MP, Hamm C, Duiverman ML, et al. Obesity hypoventilation syndrome treated with non-invasive ventilation: is a switch to CPAP therapy feasible? Respirology 2020;25(4):435–42.

32. Patout M, Dantoing E, de Marchi M, et al. Step-down from non-invasive ventilation to continuous positive airway pressure: a better phenotyping is required. Respirology 2020;25(4):456.

33. de Lucas-Ramos P, de Miguel-Díez J, Santacruz-Siminiani A, et al. Benefits at 1 year of nocturnal intermittent positive pressure ventilation in patients with obesity-hypoventi lation syndrome. Respir Med 2004;98(10):961–7.

34. Masa JF, Celli BR, Riesco JA, et al. The obesity hypoventilation syndrome can be treated with noninvasive mechanical ventilation. Chest 2001;119(4):1102–7.

35. Budweiser S, Riedl SG, Jörres RA, et al. Mortality and prognostic factors in patients with obesity-hypoventilation syndrome undergoing noninvasive ventilation. J Intern Med 2007;261(4):375–83.

36. Carrillo A, Ferrer M, Gonzalez-Diaz G, et al. Noninvasive ventilation in acute hypercapnic respiratory failure caused by obesity hypoventilation syndrome and chronic obstructive pulmonary disease. AJRCCM 2012;186(12):1279–85.

37. McNicholas WT. Impact of sleep in COPD. Chest 2000;117(2 Suppl):48S–53S.

38. Couillard A, Prefaut C. From muscle disuse to myopathy in COPD: potential contribution of oxidative stress. Eur Respir J 2005;26(4):703–19.

39. DeMarco FJJ, Wynne JW, Block AJ, et al. Oxygen desaturation during sleep as a determinant of the "Blue and Bloated" syndrome. Chest 1981;79(6):621–5.

40. Cormick W, Olson LG, Hensley MJ, et al. Nocturnal hypoxaemia and quality of sleep in patients with chronic obstructive lung disease. Thorax 1986;41(11):846–54.

41. Teodorescu M, Xie A, Sorkness CA, et al. Effects of inhaled fluticasone on upper airway during sleep and wakefulness in asthma: a pilot study. JCSM 2014;10(2):183–93.

42. Lacedonia D, Carpagnano GE, Patricelli G, et al. Prevalence of comorbidities in patients with obstructive sleep apnea syndrome, overlap syndrome and obesity hypoventilation syndrome. Clin Respir J 2018;12(5):1905–11.

43. Shawon MSR, Perret JL, Senaratna C v, et al. Current evidence on prevalence and clinical outcomes of co-morbid obstructive sleep apnea and chronic obstructive pulmonary disease: a systematic review. Sleep Med Rev 2017;32:58–68.

44. Wang Y, Hu K, Liu K, et al. Obstructive sleep apnea exacerbates airway inflammation in patients with chronic obstructive pulmonary disease. Sleep Med 2015;16(9):1123–30.

45. Tuleta I, Stöckigt F, Juergens UR, et al. Intermittent Hypoxia contributes to the lung damage by increased oxidative stress, inflammation, and Disbalance in Protease/Antiprotease system. Lung 2016;194(6):1015–20.

46. Marin JM, Soriano JB, Carrizo SJ, et al. Outcomes in patients with chronic obstructive pulmonary disease and obstructive sleep apnea: the overlap syndrome. AJRCCM 2010;182(3):325–31.

47. Chaouat A, Weitzenblum E, Krieger J, et al. Prognostic value of lung function and pulmonary haemodynamics in OSA patients treated with CPAP. Eur Respir J 1999;13(5):1091–6.

48. Petrof BJ, Kimoff RJ, Levy RD, et al. Nasal continuous positive airway pressure facilitates respiratory muscle function during sleep in severe chronic obstructive pulmonary disease. Am Rev Respir Dis 1991;143(5 Pt 1):928–35.

49. Martin JG, Shore S, Engel LA. Effect of continuous positive airway pressure on respiratory mechanics and pattern of breathing in induced asthma. Am Rev Respir Dis 1982;126(5):812–7.

50. Machado M-CL, Vollmer WM, Togeiro SM, et al. CPAP and survival in moderate-to-severe obstructive sleep apnoea syndrome and hypoxaemic COPD. Eur Respir J 2010;35(1):132–7.

51. Stanchina ML, Welicky LM, Donat W, et al. Impact of CPAP use and age on mortality in patients with combined COPD and obstructive sleep apnea: the overlap syndrome. JCSM 2013;9(8):767–72.

52. Jaoude P, Kufel T, El-Solh AA. Survival benefit of CPAP favors hypercapnic patients with the overlap syndrome. Lung 2014;192(2):251–8.

53. Ergan B, Oczkowski S, Rochwerg B, et al. European Respiratory Society guidelines on long-term home non-invasive ventilation for management of COPD. Eur Respir J 2019;54(3).

54. Macrea M, Oczkowski S, Rochwerg B, et al. Long-term noninvasive ventilation in chronic stable hypercapnic chronic obstructive pulmonary disease. An Official American thoracic society clinical practice guideline. AJRCCM 2020;202(4):e74–87.

55. Kaminska M, Rimmer KP, McKim DA, et al. Long-term non-invasive ventilation in patients with chronic obstructive pulmonary disease (COPD): 2021 Canadian Thoracic Society Clinical Practice Guideline update. Can J Respir Crit Care Sleep Med 2021;5(3):160–83.

56. McEvoy RD, Pierce RJ, Hillman D, et al. Nocturnal non-invasive nasal ventilation in stable hypercapnic

COPD: a randomised controlled trial. Thorax 2009; 64(7):561–6.

57. Struik FM, Lacasse Y, Goldstein RS, et al. Nocturnal noninvasive positive pressure ventilation in stable COPD: a systematic review and individual patient data meta-analysis. Respir Med 2014;108(2): 329–37.

58. Windisch W, Vogel M, Sorichter S, et al. Normocapnia during nIPPV in chronic hypercapnic COPD reduces subsequent spontaneous PaCO2. Respir Med 2002;96(8):572–9.

59. Windisch W, Kostić S, Dreher M, et al. Outcome of patients with stable COPD receiving controlled noninvasive positive pressure ventilation aimed at a maximal reduction of Pa(CO2). Chest 2005; 128(2):657–62.

60. Köhnlein T, Windisch W, Köhler D, et al. Non-invasive positive pressure ventilation for the treatment of severe stable chronic obstructive pulmonary disease: a prospective, multicentre, randomised, controlled clinical trial. Lancet Respir Med 2014; 2(9):698–705.

61. Struik FM, Sprooten RTM, Kerstjens HAM, et al. Nocturnal non-invasive ventilation in COPD patients with prolonged hypercapnia after ventilatory support for acute respiratory failure: a randomised, controlled, parallel-group study. Thorax 2014;69(9): 826–34.

62. Murphy PB, Rehal S, Arbane G, et al. Effect of home noninvasive ventilation with oxygen therapy vs oxygen therapy alone on hospital readmission or death after an acute COPD exacerbation: a randomized clinical trial. JAMA 2017;317(21):2177–86.

63. Duiverman ML, Maagh P, Magnet FS, et al. Impact of High-Intensity-NIV on the heart in stable COPD: a randomised cross-over pilot study. Respir Res 2017;18(1):76.

64. Tuggey JM, Plant PK, Elliott MW. Domiciliary non-invasive ventilation for recurrent acidotic exacerbations of COPD: an economic analysis. Thorax 2003;58(10):867–71.

65. Finder JD, Birnkrant D, Carl J, et al. Respiratory care of the patient with Duchenne muscular dystrophy: ATS consensus statement. AJRCCm 2004;170(4): 456–65.

66. Baydur A, Layne E, Aral H, et al. Long term non-invasive ventilation in the community for patients with musculoskeletal disorders: 46 year experience and review. Thorax 2000;55(1):4–11.

67. Lechtzin N, Scott Y, Busse AM, et al. Early use of non-invasive ventilation prolongs survival in subjects with ALS. Amyotroph Lateral Scler 2007;8(3):185–8.

68. Haverkamp LJ, Appel V, Appel SH. Natural history of amyotrophic lateral sclerosis in a database population. Validation of a scoring system and a model for survival prediction. Brain 1995;118(Pt 3):707–19.

69. Miller RG, Jackson CE, Kasarskis EJ, et al. Practice parameter update: the care of the patient with amyotrophic lateral sclerosis: drug, nutritional, and respiratory therapies (an evidence-based review): report of the Quality Standards Subcommittee of the American Academy of Neurology. Neurology 2009;73(15): 1218–26.

70. McKim DA, Road J, Avendano M, et al. Home mechanical ventilation: a Canadian Thoracic Society clinical practice guideline. Can Respir J 2011; 18(4):197–215.

71. Rimmer KP, Kaminska M, Nonoyama M, et al. Home mechanical ventilation for patients with Amyotrophic Lateral Sclerosis: a Canadian Thoracic Society clinical practice guideline. Can J Respir Crit Care Sleep Med 2019;3(1):9–27.

72. Boentert M. Sleep disturbances in patients with amyotrophic lateral sclerosis: current perspectives. Nat Sci Sleep 2019;11:97–111.

73. Patout M, Lhuillier E, Kaltsakas G, et al. Long-term survival following initiation of home non-invasive ventilation: a European study. Thorax 2020;75(11): 965–73.

74. Soudon P, Steens M, Toussaint M. A comparison of invasive versus noninvasive full-time mechanical ventilation in Duchenne muscular dystrophy. Chronic Respir Dis 2008;5(2):87–93.

75. Dhand R, Johnson JC. Care of the chronic tracheostomy. Respir Care 2006;51(9):984.

76. Struik FM, Duiverman ML, Meijer PM, et al. Volume-targeted versus pressure-targeted noninvasive ventilation in patients with chest-wall deformity: a pilot study. Respir Care 2011;56(10):1522–5.

77. Uccelli S, Pini L, Bottone D, et al. Dyspnea during night-time and at early Morning in patients with stable COPD is associated with supine tidal expiratory flow limitation. Int J chronic obstructive Pulm Dis 2020;15:2549–58.

78. Milesi I, Porta R, Cacciatore S, et al. Effects of automatic tailoring of positive end expiratory pressure (PEEP) by forced oscillation technique (FOT) during nocturnal non-invasive ventilation (NIV) in chronic obstructive pulmonary disease (COPD). Eur Respir J 2017;50(suppl 61):PA2179.

79. Vasconcelos RS, Sales RP, Melo LH de P, et al. Influences of duration of inspiratory Effort, respiratory mechanics, and ventilator Type on asynchrony with pressure support and Proportional assist ventilation. Respir Care 2017;62(5):550–7.

80. Patout M, Gagnadoux F, Rabec C, et al. AVAPS-AE versus ST mode: a randomized controlled trial in patients with obesity hypoventilation syndrome. Respirology 2020;25(10):1073–81.

81. Oscroft NS, Chadwick R, Davies MG, et al. Volume assured versus pressure preset non-invasive ventilation for compensated ventilatory failure in COPD. Respir Med 2014;108(10):1508–15.

# Best Predictors of Continuous Positive Airway Pressure Adherence

Terri E. Weaver, PhD, RN, ATSF, FAASM[a,b],*

## KEYWORDS

- Continuous positive airway pressure (CPAP) • Adherence • Compliance • PAP
- Predictors of adherence

## KEY POINTS

- There is no consistent definition of continuous positive airway pressure (CPAP) adherence, limiting the interpretation of the literature exploring potential predictors of use.
- Operative factors may differ with regards to initial acceptance of CPAP versus long-term use.
- Residual events, nasal volume, Black race (although this likely is indicative of other socioeconomic factors to be determined), use in the first 2 weeks of treatment, active and planful problem solving, and claustrophobic tendencies seem to be the "best" predictors of CPAP use.
- Conflicting support exists for the role of several factors that represent disease pathophysiology, clinical features, demographic characteristics, device-related variables, and psychological factors.
- The effect size of statistically significant differences associated with salient variables in addition to understanding the role of phenotypes in CPAP acceptance requires further investigation.

## BACKGROUND

Continuous positive airway pressure (CPAP) currently is the most effective treatment of obstructive sleep apnea (OSA) providing a pneumatic splint that stabilizes the upper airway preventing full or partial collapse during sleep. Although the efficacy of this treatment has been well established through randomized clinical trials, its effectiveness, or application in the real world of clinical practice, is hampered by decreased acceptance with rates of 29% to 83% for use <4 h/night rising to 46% to 83% for use less than 4.5 h/night.[1] These rates of adherence are similar to adherence profiles for other chronic diseases such as asthma and home oxygen therapy.[2] Nevertheless, CPAP adherence in OSA is critical to reducing comorbidities associated with OSA such as cardiovascular disease, hypertension, diabetes, as well as improving quality of life,

reducing neurocognitive impairment, mood, accidents, and impact on overall mortality.[3–6] Indeed, after 1 year of treatment, mortality for those non-adherent to CPAP is almost 2 times greater than who are adherent.[6] Consistent with chronic disease management, gaining an understanding of why patients don't adhere to treatment will enhance the approach to care delivery, promote personalized health care and the development of effective interventions to facilitate treatment use. This article reviews factors in the literature, especially in the last 10 years, \ that have been shown to be instrumental in the patient's use of CPAP with an emphasis on the best predictors.

One of the challenges in addressing CPAP adherence is defining the "dose." There is no consensus on the prescription for nightly use.[4] This makes it difficult to establish goals when the treatment objective is ill-defined. Weaver and

[a] College of Nursing, University of Illinois Chicago, 814 Franklin AvenueRiver Forest, IL 60305, USA; [b] School of Nursing, University of Pennsylvania
* College of Nursing, University of Illinois Chicago.
E-mail address: teweaver@uic.edu

Sleep Med Clin 17 (2022) 587–595
https://doi.org/10.1016/j.jsmc.2022.07.005
1556-407X/22/© 2022 Elsevier Inc. All rights reserved.

coinvestigators suggested that the "dose" or nightly use may be dependent on the aim of treatment.[7] Different cut points or "doses" were evident depending on whether the metric was improvement in subjectively measured daytime sleepiness, which may be a patient aspiration; reduced objectively measured daytime sleepiness as would be applied in occupation safety situations; or overall enhancement of quality of life, the overall purpose of health care.[7] For those who had an Epworth Sleepiness Scale (ESS) score of less than 11, $\geq$ 4 hour/night was sufficient to obtain a normal value.[7] Longer use was required to have an impact on objectively measured sleepiness (MSLT), whereby 6 hours/night was required, and 7.5 hours/night was necessary to produce optimal benefit to quality of life as measured by the Functional Outcomes of Sleep Questionnaire (FOSQ).[7] Kribbs and colleagues were one of the first to attempt to define CPAP adherence applying an *a priori* definition of at least 4 hours, 70% of the nights.[8] This definition, applied by the Centers for Medicare and Medicaid Services (CMS),[9] has been embraced by the field and used as the predominant definition in the literature to define CPAP adherence. Actually, the correlation between nightly hours of use and proportion of nights used is quite high (rho = $-0.73$) as those who have high hours of nightly use also use apply CPAP more frequently, so the hourly reference alone may be sufficient.[10]

Taking a different approach, other investigators have used categorical definitions to define adherence such as <2h, 2–6h, and greater than 6 h per night[11] or created thresholds such as greater than 5 or > 7 h/night.[12] Conditional definitions were also used to characterize the type of adherence. For example, van Zeller and associates classified CPAP nightly use as very good greater than 90% of days and >6 h/night, good within the range of 70% to 90% of the days and > 4 h/night, and poor if it was lower less than 70% of the days and <4 h/night.[2] Objection to these approaches is the reliance on device determined length of use without the context of sleep duration. Certainly, a patient may use CPAP 4 hr./night during either 4 or 8 hours of sleep duration, and hence the assessment of being adherent would change accordingly. Acknowledging this, Fujita and coworkers as well as others have advocated for a definition that incorporates sleep duration.[4,13] In addition to the > 4 h/night for greater than 70% of the nights, they used an "enhanced" definition of greater than 80% of self-reported sleep duration.[13] The move toward personalized health care dictates that whether a patient is considered adherent depends on the response to treatment

as some patients do well with less nightly use than others.[7] In this determination, Bakker and co-authors suggest that there be consideration of the sensitivity of the outcome measure used to evaluate response to treatment, the level of impairment pretreatment, and hours of habitual sleep duration relative to nightly device use.[4]

## INDEPENDENT PREDICTORS OF CONTINUOUS POSITIVE AIRWAY PRESSURE ADHERENCE

Exploration of reasons why some patients are more adherent than others has considered several distinct variables in independent associations. These have included variables related to the mask interface and type of device as well as initial use, demographic variables, physiologic variables including disease severity and symptoms, comorbidities, and psychological factors. Unfortunately, these analyses have not yielded the silver bullet that we seek, but they do help to paint a picture of who may be at high risk for nonadherence and those considerations that are most operative. It should be noted that although these associations are important, in themselves, they fail to consider all potential influences that may be equally or more in effect or interact to diminish or enhance adherence.

### Mask Interface

It goes without saying, that if you do not wear a mask, you do not experience side effects associated with its use. Although 34% of patients report mask-related side effects, early studies have shown that the technological interface does not influence treatment adherence.[10,14] Indeed, Ulander and associates found that CPAP side effects, most mask related, did not differentiate those who continued to use CPAP and those who discontinued treatment.[15] For the most part, investigations have centered around the comparison of mask type that most promote CPAP use. Some studies found that the nasal mask promotes higher use than nasal pillows, full face mask, or oronasal mask while others reported no difference between interfaces.[16–21] One review of studies evaluating the impact of different types of masks on treatment efficacy and adherence concluded that the performance of oronasal masks was inferior to nasal masks in addition to reduced adherence with 1 hour less nightly device use.[22] There was similarity in efficacy and adherence between nasal masks and pillows.[22] Advances in mask design have provided patients with greater options and enabling patients to be highly involved in mask selection should be a priority in care of these patients. Moreover, although general mask type does not influence adherence, for specific issues such as leaks and mouth breathing, certain masks may be more effective.[21]

### Device-Related Factors

Variables associated with the device that might affect adherence include set pressure, presence of leaks, residual events (AHI), and use of humidi-fication. Although CPAP manufacturers have developed devices with pressure control capabilities such as autoPAP, ramp, or flexible pressure with the conviction that pressure influences adherence, the predominance of evidence indicated this is not the case.[15,17,23–25] Mask leaks need to be addressed immediately, although they do not directly affect adherence per se. Sabil and team found that an important leak (mean % turbine time 1.7 [5.3] determined by device EncoreAny-ware software) > 60 minutes for 90 days, adversely affected adherence, but presumably such a condition would be immediately addressed and not persist for such a long period of time.[26] More to the point, leaks may be a source of residual events, which have been shown to affect treatment adherence.[27,28] Nasal congestion, most often associated with mouth breathers, has been reported in 64% of CPAP users.[21] In several studies, having a stuffy nose and dry mouth among other side effects has affected CPAP use, but again, the side effects are only experienced when CPAP is applied producing a weak influence on adherence.[15,24] Although humidification is routinely applied to address these types of side effects, the data in support of its use,[6,29–31] is outweighed by data that show little impact on adherence,[24,32–34] including discussion on this topic by the American Academy of Sleep Medicine.[32] Potentially contributing to the sensation of a "blocked nose" is decreased nasal volume. Indeed, there is a support that the volume of the nose, and not stuffiness, affect adherence, suggesting the importance of having an otorhinolaryngology evaluation.[24,35–37]

### Disease Severity, Daytime Sleepiness, and Function

Intuitively, disease severity, that is, the level of AHI or ODI, would play a role in the degree of adherence. However, there is limited evidence demonstrating this and those studies that have statistically reliable findings have weak associations.[21,24] For example, although Jacobsen and colleagues found statistically significant differences between disease severity levels with 54.5% adherence for mild OSA, 71.3% for moderate, and 89.1% for severe,[29] other studies were unable to produce statistically significant or robust relationships between disease severity and CPAP use.[2,15,17,23–26,38–42] Likewise, neither the oxygen saturation trough, $Pao_2$ or $Pco_2$ were factors in determining adherence.[17,40,43,44] Some investigators documented that Body Mass Index (BMI) affected adherence with those with greater BMI less adherent,[6,17,26,28,39,45] while most have not.[3,13,15,24,38,40,44] One might consider that higher BMI is not only indicative for disease severity, but also associated with increased daytime sleepiness possibly producing collineality.[46,47] For the most part, medical comorbidities do not seem to be a major factor in the tendency to adhere to CPAP treatment.[2,3,15,26,29,38,43,44]

Excessive daytime sleepiness is the predominant symptom of OSA and most often the reason for seeking medical attention. Although there is some support that pretreatment level of sleepiness influences adherence,[6,24,29,45,48,49] a greater number of studies show little relationship.[2,13,15,17,23,24,38,39,41,43,50] What seems to be more motivating is the patient perception of improvement in daytime sleepiness.[24] Similarly, a few investigations demonstrate that daily functioning/quality of life before treatment affects adherence[25,41] while others do not.[24,27,38,39,43,45] Again, perceived change in daily functioning and quality of life may be more operative than the baseline value.

### Demographic Variables - or - Things You Can't Change!

Older patients tend to be more adherent than younger patients, but this is not a robust or consistent associaiton.[2,3,6,13,15,23–26,29,38–40,43–45] One study reported that for every decade increase in age, CPAP use increased by 35.03 minutes (95% CI, 13.47–56.58 min), an increase that may not be clinically meaningful.[38] Sex also does not seem to be differential with regard to adherence.[6,13,15,17,23–26,29,38–40,43,45,50] A caveat is that most study participants were predominantly male, reflective of disease prevalence, reducing the heterogeneity of these investigations and potential to detect differences.

For reasons that remain unclear, several studies have shown that African Americans use CPAP less than Whites, with a difference of almost 2 hours.[21,23,24,27,41,44,51–53] This difference is a notable predictor of use during the first week of treatment and is still present 6 months later.[27,44] In fact, May and coworkers found that in exploring predictors of treatment use, race was a factor that remained in the prediction model until use in the first week was added.[38] Indeed, Schwartz and colleagues reported that at 2 weeks of treatment, 26% of African Americans and 47% of Whites used CPAP $\geq$ 4 h/night 70% of nights and at 6 months, 33% African Americans and 47% Whites met this criterion, which was statistically reliable.[44] These disparities persisted when the model was adjusted for differences in demographic variables, median income, and/or comorbidity.[44] However, African Americans with more severe disease were three times more likely to use CPAP than those with mild or moderate disease.[44] Schwartz and coauthors note that this health inequity is not isolated to CPAP treatment as adherence to screenings and medication adherence differs between African Americans and Whites in other illnesses.[44] In a comparison of device application between White, African American, and Hispanic CPAP-treated patients, Diaz-Abad and colleagues found no difference in use among the 3 race/ethic groups both in terms of hours per night, number of days per week and $\geq$ 4 hr./night 70% nights, although it should be pointed out that hours of use was self-reported and not based on the objective data.[41]

Health inequities are multifactorial, but may be linked to socioeconomic status whereby income, difficulty accessing health care, local resources represented by zip code, obtaining child care, and health literacy may be play a role.[21,53,54] This was illustrated by Platt and coworkers who found differences in adherence by zip code after adjusting for socioeconomic factors and comorbidity with use $\geq$4 h/night in lower economic zip codes of 34.1% compared with 62.3% in zip codes of higher economic status.[54] To the point, in their investigation, Billings and team found that race, education, and ZIP code were highly correlated.[53] In their comparison of CPAP use between Māori and non-Māori populations, Bakker and coauthors discovered, unlike others,[21] that income was not as much of a factor in differences in use as was patient report of deprivation.[23] Others have also reported that income was not a factor in adherence.[38,43,44] But, being used, especially as an occupational driver, and having a professional position versus blue collar job produced higher use.[40,43,50] Moreover, although having tertiary education was a factor in one study, health literacy was not.[23] Education level did not seem to affect adherence in other studies.[15,43,44,55] For Hispanic patients and those whereby English is a second language, spoken language between patient and provider was not a barrier to being adherent.[41]

The influence of the patient's partner on adherence can be a mixed bag. As one might surmise, it is dependent on the overall positivity and nature of the relationship. Hoy and coworkers demonstrated that CPAP use was significantly less at 1, 3, and 6 months if the patient was referred for treatment by their partner rather than self-referred.[56] After interviewing 20 couples, Ye and colleagues reported that facilitators to CPAP use were whether the partner aided in the diagnosis and treatment, they worked together to cope with having OSA, both patient and partner perceived the benefit of CPAP treatment, the patient desiring to use CPAP to benefit the partner, and if the partner provided support to the patient to use CPAP.[57] However, this group also indicated that barriers to use were if the couples had anxiety about CPAP treatment, the equipment was viewed as bothersome and disruptive of both the patient and the partner's sleep, affecting intimacy, and the patient was embarrassed or viewed as unattractive when wearing the mask.[57] The partner's engagement not only affects disease-specific quality of life, but the quality of the marriage was found to be an intervening variable with examining the relationship between partner engagement and CPAP adherence.[58] However, despite this salient descriptive data, marital status as a demographic has not been a predictor of CPAP adherence.[2,13,24]

## Psychological factors - or - things you can change

### Self-Efficacy
There is fairly compelling data that initial use of CPAP predicts long-term use.[2,38,39,50] Indeed, Turnbull and associates found that 50% of the variance in long-term use was explained by use in the first 2 to 4 weeks of treatment.[39] Moreover, the decision whether to use CPAP is made by the fourth day of treatment.[10] This vulnerable time period is when perceptions or cognitions about the treatment are formed, or more the case, formed before CPAP treatment. Cognitions related to health behaviors include the perceptions of risk of the illness, benefit of the treatment (outcome expectancies), and volition or self-efficacy to engage in the desired behavior.[59] Collectively, these 3 cognitions are known as self-efficacy.[59] Ye and coinvestigators reported that although the perception of risk, outcome expectancies, and treatment self-efficacy were not associated with adherence before treatment initiation, treatment self-efficacy was significantly associated with adherence during the first week of treatment, suggesting that early exposure to CPAP influences beliefs.[27] Indeed, in one study patients expressed knowledge of the benefits of CPAP, less than half believed that they could overcome the barrier to using CPAP if it made them feel

claustrophobic or disturbed their bedpartner's sleep.[59] Although the evidence indicating that self-efficacy is an independent predictor of treatment use is mixed,[17,21,23–25,38,41] as Crawford points out, self-efficacy in combination with models such as social cognitive theory, health belief, health locus of control, transtheoretical model and stage/readiness for change, account for 11% to 58% of the variance in CPAP use and have the greatest utility when measured posttreatment.[24] Stepnowsky and others have found that the traits of active coping, planful problem solving and the willingness to troubleshoot difficulties with therapy, were more likely to be adherent to CPAP.[21,60]

### Claustrophobic Tendencies

The tendency toward claustrophobia is a deterrent to CPAP use.[61,62] Those who used CPAP less than 2 h/night had higher scores on a modified measure of claustrophobia and agoraphobia (Fear and Avoidance Scale [FAAS]) and these scores were less likely to change over time.[61] However, those with higher levels of use had a significant change in FAAS score from pre to posttreatment, indicating acclamation to the therapy.[61] Pretreatment claustrophobic tendencies were found in 15% of patients with sleep apnea, but in another study after one night of treatment that proportion was 63% with 44% of men and 84% women and was predictive of both short and long-term nonadherence.[61,62]

### Mood

Some have explored whether psychological factors such as anxiety, depression, or personality traits affect adherence.[24–26,28,38,43,50] Except for isolated studies, anxiety, and depression as well as personality disorders don't seem to have an important influence on adherence.[13,24,26,38,50]

## PREDICTORS IN MULTIVARIATE ANALYSES

A limitation of much of the work on CPAP adherence is the utilization of univariate analyses, which incorporates a limited exploration of potential factors, interactions, and relative weight. This weakness is likely related to the large sample size that would be required to perform multiple variate analyses with sufficient power to detect differences.

In multivariable analyses, Law and colleagues examined variables that might affect adherence during CPAP titration.[28] A 3-factor final regression model consisting of $SpO_2$, depression, lower 95th percentile pressure that was based on univariate analyses, explained 18.5% of autoPAP use.[28] Considering the first week of treatment, salient

predictors in the final model for this time period in another study included Black race, residual events, and whether CPAP affected intimacy.[27] After univariate analyses that included demographic variables, AHI, BMI, ESS, sustained attention, and quality of life, Turnbull and associates applied linear regression to significant factors for long-term use.[39] Forward multivariate analysis selected gender and backwards analysis indicated both gender and BMI and although gender was foremost, it explained very little of the variance in CPAP use.[39] Examining socio-demographic, AHI, leak, pressure, self-efficacy, social support, anxiety, depression, family coping, and quality of life, the final model in Sampaio and coworker's study included age, quality of life, family coping (with an interaction), decisional balance and cognitive representations, and time that explained use at 6 months of treatment.[25] Participants with a higher self-efficacy were twice as likely to be adherent and family coping was only associated with adherence when self-efficacy was in the model together producing an odds ratio of 17.443.[25] Looking at social variables, Billings and coinvestigators tested the potential predictors of AHI, ESS, gender, pressure level, marital status, smoking, race/ethnicity, education, employment, and socioeconomic status by zip code for use at 1 and 3 months.[53] Race was the only predictor for use in the first month, but at 3 months, it remained in the model only when socioeconomic status was adjusted accounting for 6% to 12% of the variance.[53] Having a home sleep test and an AHI greater than 62 were the only other variables that remained in the final model.[53] Palm and partners found that in logistic regression female gender and the presence of hypertension were factors in nonadherence, but age, more severe disease, higher ESS, and using a humidifier reduced the risk of discontinuing treatment, suggesting that different variables may be at play with regard to initiating and sustaining use.[6] In a Japanese population, Tanahashi and collaborators conducted multivariate analyses that included variables from the titration night, clinical variables such as EKG, and blood gases, disease severity, socioeconomic factors, gender, comorbidities, depression, and occupation. This testing yielded a final model that comprised being an occupational driver, bedtime, subjective sleep quality, sleep efficiency during titration, and positive attitude toward CPAP significantly predictive of adherence.[43] Including a host of variables such as age, gender, disease severity, BMI, BP, cholesterol, comorbidities, statin use, and major adverse cardiac and cerebral events (MACCE), the Cox analysis final model presented by Baratta and team contained

**Table 1**
**Classification of potential predictors based on the predominance of evidence**

| "Best" Predictors | Conflicting Evidence | Not Predictive |
|---|---|---|
| Residual apneic and hypopneic events[27,28] | Disease severity (AHI; disease classification, oxygenation)[2,15,17,21,23–26,29,38–44] | Mask and technological interface[10,14,15] |
| Nasal volume[24,35–37] | BMI[3,6,13,15,17,24,26,28,38–40,44,45] | Pressure setting[15,17,23–25] |
| Black race[21,23,24,27,41,44,51–53] | Pretreatment daytime sleepiness & quality of life[2,6,13,15,17,23,24,29,38,39,41,43,45,48–50] | CPAP side effects[15,24] |
| Use in first 2 weeks of treatment[2,38,39,50] | Older age[2,3,6,13,15,23–26,29,38–40,43–45] | Medical comorbidities[2,3,15,26,29,38,43,44] |
| Active and planful problem solving[21,60] | Humidification[6,24,29–34] | Sex[6,13,15,17,23–26,29,38–40,43,45,51] |
| Claustrophobic tendency[61,62] | Partner relationship[2,13,24,57,58] | Income[21,23,38,43,44] |
| | Self-efficacy[17,21,23–25,27,38,41] | Health literacy[23] and education[15,43,44,55] |
| | | Anxiety, depression, and personality disorders[13,24,26,38,50] |

lower OSA severity, cigarette smoking, and MACCE as independent predictors of long-term nonadherence controlling for age, gender, and metabolic syndrome.[3]

## SUMMARY

There is not one variable that is the best predictor of CPAP adherence (**Table 1**). It is likely that there are many factors that influence CPAP nightly use and may differ depending on whether you want to promote initial acceptance or long-term adherence. It seems that patient readiness to use the treatment and their perceptions regarding the impact of OSA on their health and their belief they can apply the treatment to achieve benefits they can articulate does affect early use. Indeed, if it is the patient's or medical provider's idea to seek treatment, acceptance is more likely than if it is the partner's suggestion.[56]

Long-term use is related to use in the first weeks of treatment, so intervention needs to be concentrated during this time. Thus, the investment both in terms of the health team as well as family to support the patient will be essential in moving a tentative patient forward to treatment acceptance. Follow-up during the first week of treatment to assess perceptions, coach, encourage, and troubleshooting is essential. This is emphasized by the fact that interventions to promote CPAP use

based on perception and cognitions seem to be most effective.[63,64]

Black race seems to be critical to initial acceptance as well as long-term use, although it is likely reflective of other operating influences. The underpinning for racial differences is likely aligned with health disparities observed in health care delivery and treatment. Assumptions should not be made about who will adhere to treatment merely based on race. Indeed, approaches to disease management should be individualized. Although health literacy has not been demonstrated to be a major factor, it may be that health literacy in combination with income, education level, and access to health care are influential.

Most studies have involved univariate analyses restricting the full understanding of the most active variable(s) given the consideration of other factors. There have been a few multi-variable regression analyses, but few state the power associated with their study. Failure to state the power associated with an investigation makes it difficult to discern whether nonsignificant findings are truly statistically unreliable or a Type II error. Moreover, there is a dearth of information regarding effect sizes related to detected differences. Although differences may be significant, without stating the effect size, the magnitude of the impact and whether it is clinically meaningful is unclear. This limitation should be addressed in future studies.

Several phenotypes have been proposed for OSA, predominantly categorized based on risk factor/environmental, clinical, pathophysiologic, biologic, genomic/genetic) features.[65] There has been little examination of outcomes linked to the proposed phenotypes including treatment adherence.[65] In addition to the continued pursuit of factors associated with CPAP use, the role of phenotypes as predictors of adherence should also be explored. In summary, do we know what the best predictors of CPAP adherence are? No, not quite, but we are getting close!

## DISCLOSURE

The author receives royalty fees for use of the Functional Outcomes of Sleep Questionnaire (FOSQ) from the following corporations: Philips Respironics, Nyxoah, Bayer AG, ResMed Germany, Jazz Pharmaceuticals, Cook Medical, RWS; Verily Life Sciences; Stratevi; LivaNova; Valis Biosciences Inc.; Clinical Outcomes Solutions; Eli Lilly; Signant Health; Signifier Medical Technologies; Harmony Biosciences; Alkermes, Syneos; Ignes Therapeutics; Takeda Development Center Americas, Inc.; and Axsome. The author is a consultant for Bayer AG, Eli Lilly, Idorsia Alliance for Sleep, and Alkermes Orexin Advisory Board.

## CLINICS CARE POINTS

- Adherence is established in the first week of treatment.

- Most perceptions of CPAP are formed prior to treatment, so understanding the patient's treatment perceptions is important in developing interventions to promote adherence.

- Patient cognitions regarding OSA and CPAP are more influential than disease severity, mask interface, nasal stuffieness or CPAP pressure level.

- Partners should be inlcuded in education sessions about CPAP.

- Patients should be given the ability to select their own equipment that will promote comfort and use.6. Assessment for claustrophobic tendencies prior to or upon initiation of CPAP could identify the need for other interventions to promote use.

## REFERENCES

1. Weaver TE, Grunstein RR. Adherence to continuous positive airway pressure therapy: the challenge to effective treatment. Proc Am Thorac Soc 2008;5(2): 173–8.

2. van Zeller M, Severo M, Santos AC, et al. 5-Years APAP adherence in OSA patients – do first impressions matter? Respir Med 2013;107(12):2046–52.

3. Baratta F, Pastori D, Bucci T, et al. Long-term prediction of adherence to continuous positive air pressure therapy for the treatment of moderate/severe obstructive sleep apnea syndrome. Sleep Med 2018;43:66–70.

4. Bakker JP, Weaver TE, Parthasarathy S, et al. Adherence to CPAP: what should we be aiming for, and how can we get there? Chest 2019;155(6):1272–87.

5. Weaver TE, Mancini C, Maislin G, et al. Continuous positive airway pressure treatment of sleepy patients with milder obstructive sleep apnea. Results of the CPAP Apnea Trial North American Program (CATNAP) Randomized Clinical Trial. Am J Resp Crit Care Med 2012;186(7):677–83.

6. Palm A, Midgren B, Theorell-Haglöw J, et al. Factors influencing adherence to continuous positive airway pressure treatment in obstructive sleep apnea and mortality associated with treatment failure – a national registry-based cohort study. Sleep Med 2018;51:85–91.

7. Weaver TE, Maislin G, Dinges DF, et al. Relationship between hours of CPAP use and achieving normal levels of sleepiness and daily functioning. Sleep 2007;30(6):711–9.

8. Kribbs NB, Pack AI, Kline LR, et al. Objective measurement of patterns of nasal CPAP use by patients with obstructive sleep apnea. Am Rev Respir Dis 1993;147(4):887–95.

9. Centers for Medicare and Medicaid Services. National Coverage determination (NCD) for durable medical equipment reference list (280.1). 2005. Available at: https://www.cms.gov/medicare-coverage-database/details/ncd-details.aspx?NCDId=190. Accessed October 10, 2021.

10. Weaver TE, Kribbs NB, Pack AI, et al. Night-to-night variability in CPAP use over the first three months of treatment. Sleep 1997;20(4):278–83.

11. Zimmerman ME, Arnedt JT, Stanchina M, et al. Normalization of memory performance and positive airway pressure adherence in memory-impaired patients with obstructive sleep apnea. Chest 2006; 130(6):1772–8.

12. Antic NA, Catcheside P, McEvoy RD, et al. The Effect of CPAP in normalizing daytime sleepiness, quality of life, and neurocognitive function in patients with moderate to severe OSA. Sleep 2011;34(1):111–9.

13. Fujita Y, Yamauchi M, Uyama H, et al. Variability of breathing during wakefulness while using CPAP predicts adherence. Respirology 2017;22(2):386–93.

14. Drake CL, Day R, Hudgel D, et al. Sleep during titration predicts continuous positive airway pressure compliance. Sleep 2003;26(3):308–11.

15. Ulander M, Johansson MS, Ewaldh AE, et al. Side effects to continuous positive airway pressure treatment for obstructive sleep apnoea: changes over time and association to adherence. Sleep & Breath 2014;18(4):799–807.

16. Massie CA, Hart RW. Clinical outcomes related to interface type in patients with obstructive sleep apnea/hypopnea syndrome who are using continuous positive airway pressure. Chest 2003;123(4): 1112–8.

17. Zampogna E, Spanevello A, Lucioni AM, et al. Adherence to continuous positive airway pressure in patients with obstructive sleep apnoea. A ten year real life study. Resp Med 2019;150:95–100.

18. Anderson FE, Kingshott RN, Taylor DR, et al. A randomized crossover efficacy trial of oral CPAP (oracle) compared with nasal CPAP in the management of obstructive sleep apnea. Sleep 2003;26(6): 721–6.

19. Beecroft J, Zanon S, Lukic D, et al. Oral continuous positive airway pressure for sleep apnea: effectiveness, patient preference, and adherence. Chest 2003;124(6):2200–8.

20. Khanna R, Kline LR. A prospective 8 week trial of nasal interfaces vs. a novel oral interface (Oracle™) for treatment of obstructive sleep apnea hypopnea syndrome. Sleep Med 2003;4(4):333–8.

21. Mehrtash M, Bakker JP, Ayas N. Predictors of continuous positive airway pressure adherence in patients with obstructive sleep apnea. Lung 2019;197(2): 115–21.

22. Andrade RG, Piccin VS, Nascimento JA, et al. Impact of the type of mask on the effectiveness of and adherence to continuous positive airway pressure treatment for obstructive sleep apnea. Jornal brasileiro de pneumologia 2014;40(6):658–68.

23. Bakker JP, O'Keeffe KM, Neill AM, et al. Ethnic disparities in CPAP adherence in New Zealand: effects of socioeconomic status, health literacy and self-efficacy. Sleep 2011;34(11):1595–603.

24. Crawford MR, Espie CA, Bartlett DJ, et al. Integrating psychology and medicine in CPAP adherence – new concepts? Sleep Med Rev 2013;18(2): 123–39.

25. Sampaio R, Pereira MG, Winck JC. Obstructive sleep apnea representations, self-efficacy and family coping regarding APAP adherence: a longitudinal study. Psych, Health Med 2014;19(1):59–69.

26. Sabil A, Le Vaillant M, Stitt C, et al. A CPAP data-based algorithm for automatic early prediction of therapy adherence. Sleep & Breath. 2021;25(2): 957–62.

27. Ye L, Pack AI, Maislin G, et al. Predictors of continuous positive airway pressure use during the first week of treatment. J Seep Res 2012;21(4):419–26.

28. Law M, Naughton M, Ho S, et al. Depression may reduce adherence during CPAP titration trial. J Clin Sleep Med 2014;10(2):163–9.

29. Jacobsen AR, Eriksen F, Hansen RW, et al. Determinants for adherence to continuous positive airway pressure therapy in obstructive sleep apnea. PLoS One 2017;12(12). e0189614-e0189614.

30. Massie CA, Hart RW, Peralez K, et al. Effects of humidification on nasal symptoms and compliance in sleep apnea patients using continuous positive airway pressure. Chest 1999;116(2):403–8.

31. Neill AM, Wai HS, Bannan SP, et al. Humidified nasal continuous positive airway pressure in obstructive sleep apnoea. Eur Respir J 2003;22(2):258–62.

32. Patil SP, Ayappa IA, Caples SM, et al. Treatment of adult obstructive sleep apnea with positive airway pressure: an American Academy of Sleep Medicine Clinical Practice Guideline. J Clin Sleep Med 2019; 15(2):335–43.

33. Duong M, Jayaram L, Camfferman D, et al. Use of heated humidification during nasal CPAP titration in obstructive sleep apnoea syndrome. Eur Respir J 2005;26(4):679–85.

34. Mador MJ, Krauza M, Pervez A, et al. Effect of heated humidification on compliance and quality of life in patients with sleep apnea using nasal continuous positive airway pressure. Chest 2005;128(4): 2151–8.

35. Li HY, Engleman H, Hsu CY, et al. Acoustic reflection for nasal airway measurement in patients with obstructive sleep apnea-hypopnea syndrome. Sleep 2005;28(12):1554–9.

36. Sugiura T, Noda A, Nakata S, et al. Influence of nasal resistance on initial acceptance of continuous positive airway pressure in treatment for obstructive sleep apnea syndrome. Respiration 2007;74(1): 56–60.

37. Morris LG, Setlur J, Burschtin OE, et al. Acoustic rhinometry predicts tolerance of nasal continuous positive airway pressure: a pilot study. Am J Rhinol 2006;20(2):133–7.

38. May AM, Gharibeh T, Wang L, et al. CPAP Adherence Predictors in a randomized trial of moderate-to-severe OSA enriched with women and minorities. Chest 2018;154(3):567–78.

39. Turnbull CD, Bratton DJ, Craig SE, et al. In patients with minimally symptomatic OSA can baseline characteristics and early patterns of CPAP usage predict those who are likely to be longer-term users of CPAP. J Thorac Dis 2016;8(2):276–81.

40. Alves C, Caminha JMPC, da Silva AM, et al. Compliance to continuous positive airway pressure therapy in a group of Portuguese patients with obstructive sleep apnea syndrome. Sleep and Breath 2012; 16(2):555–62.

41. Diaz-Abad M, Chatila W, Lammi MR, et al. Determinants of CPAP adherence in Hispanics with obstructive sleep apnea. Sleep Dis 2014;2014:878213–6.

42. Wolkove N, Baltzan M, Kamel H, et al. Long-term compliance with continuous positive airway pressure in patients with obstructive sleep apnea. Can Respir J 2008;15(7):365–9.

43. Tanahashi T, Nagano J, Yamaguchi Y, et al. Factors that predict adherence to continuous positive airway pressure treatment in obstructive sleep apnea patients: a prospective study in Japan. Sleep and Biolog Rhythms 2012;10(2):126–35.

44. Schwartz SW, Sebastião Y, Rosas J, et al. Racial disparity in adherence to positive airway pressure among US veterans. Sleep & Breath 2016;20(3):947–55.

45. Nadal N, de Batlle J, Barbé F, et al. Predictors of CPAP compliance in different clinical settings: primary care versus sleep unit. Sleep and Breath 2018;22(1):157–63.

46. Vgontzas AN, Bixler EO, Tan TL, et al. Obesity without sleep apnea is associated with daytime sleepiness. Arch Intern Med 1998;158(12):1333–7.

47. Romero-Corral A, Caples SM, Lopez-Jimenez F, et al. Interactions between Obesity and obstructive sleep apnea: Implications for treatment. Chest 2010;137(3):711–9.

48. McArdle N, Devereux G, Heidarnejad H, et al. Long-term use of CPAP therapy for sleep apnea/hypopnea syndrome. Am J Respir Crit Care Med 1999;159(4 Pt 1):1108–14.

49. Hollandt JH, Mahlerwein M. Nasal breathing and continuous positive airway pressure (CPAP) in patients with obstructive sleep apnea (OSA). Sleep & Breath 2003;7(2):87–93.

50. Gulati A, Ali M, Davies M, et al. A prospective observational study to evaluate the effect of social and personality factors on continuous positive airway pressure (CPAP) compliance in obstructive sleep apnoea syndrome. BMC Pulm Med 2017;17(1):56.

51. Sawyer AM, Canamucio A, Moriarty H, et al. Do cognitive perceptions influence CPAP use? Patient Educ Couns 2010;85(1):85–91.

52. Lord S, Sawyer B, O'Connell D, et al. Night-to-night variability of disturbed breathing during sleep in an elderly community sample. Sleep 1991;14(3):252–8.

53. Billings ME, Auckley D, Benca R, et al. Race and residential socioeconomics as predictors of CPAP adherence. Sleep 2011;34(12):1653–8.

54. Platt AB, Field SH, Asch DA, et al. Neighborhood of residence is associated with daily adherence to CPAP therapy. Sleep 2009;32(6):799–806.

55. Fornas C, Ballester E, Arteta E, et al. Measurement of general health status in obstructive sleep apnea hypopnea patients. Sleep 1995;18(10):876–9.

56. Hoy CJ, Vennelle M, Kingshott RN, et al. Can intensive support improve continuous positive airway pressure use in patients with the sleep apnea/hypopnea syndrome? Am J Respir Crit Care Med 1999;159(4 Pt 1):1096–100.

57. Ye L, Antonelli MT, Willis DG, et al. Couples' experiences with continuous positive airway pressure treatment: a dyadic perspective. Sleep Health 2017;3(5):362–7.

58. Gentina T, Bailly S, Jounieaux F, et al. Marital quality, partner's engagement and continuous positive airway pressure adherence in obstructive sleep apnea. Sleep Med 2019;55:56–61.

59. Weaver TE, Maislin G, Dinges DF, et al. Self-efficacy in sleep apnea: instrument development and patient perceptions of obstructive sleep apnea risk, treatment benefit, and volition to use continuous positive airway pressure. Sleep 2003;26(6):727–32.

60. Stepnowsky CJ, Bardwell WA, Moore PJ, et al. Psychologic correlates of compliance with continuous positive airway pressure. Sleep 2002;25(7):758–62.

61. Chasens ER, Pack AI, Maislin G, et al. Claustrophobia and adherence to CPAP treatment. West J Nurs Res 2005;27(3):307–21.

62. Edmonds JC, Yang H, King T, et al. Claustrophobic tendencies and continuous positive airway pressure therapy non-adherence in adults with obstructive sleep apnea. Heart & Lung 2015;44(2):100–6.

63. Richards D, Bartlett DJ, Wong K, et al. Increased adherence to CPAP with a group cognitive behavioral treatment intervention: a randomized trial. Sleep 2007;30(5):635–40.

64. Olsen S, Smith SS, Oei TPS, et al. Motivational interviewing (MINT) improves continuous positive airway pressure (CPAP) acceptance and adherence: a randomized controlled trial. J Couns Clin Psych 2012;80(1):151–63.

65. Zinchuk AV, Gentry MJ, Concato J, et al. Phenotypes in obstructive sleep apnea: a definition, examples and evolution of approaches. Sleep Med Rev 2016;35:113–23.

# Comorbid Insomnia and Sleep Apnea
## Assessment and Management Approaches

Alexander Sweetman, PhD[a],*, Leon Lack, PhD[b], Megan Crawford, PhD[c],
Douglas M. Wallace, MD[d,e]

## KEYWORDS

• COMISA • OSA • PAP therapy • PAP adherence • CBTi • Cognitive behavioral therapy for insomnia

## KEY POINTS

- Approximately 30% to 50% of patients with obstructive sleep apnea (OSA) in sleep clinics report comorbid insomnia symptoms.
- Patients with comorbid insomnia and sleep apnea (COMISA) have worse sleep, mental health, physical health, and quality of life, compared with patients with either insomnia or sleep apnea alone.
- Patients with COMISA use positive airway pressure (PAP) therapy for fewer hours per night, compared with patients with sleep apnea alone. Consequently, it is important to identify and manage insomnia symptoms among patients with OSA.
- Cognitive behavioral therapy for insomnia (CBTi) is recommended as the "first-line" treatment for insomnia. CBTi is an effective insomnia treatment in the presence of untreated OSA. CBTi may also reduce the severity of OSA and improve adherence to PAP therapy in patients with moderate and severe OSA.
- Many sleep clinics worldwide currently specialize in the diagnosis and management of OSA alone. Sleep clinics should incorporate insomnia assessment tools, and evidence-based insomnia treatment and referral pathways, to provide personalized care for patients with COMISA. Potential CBTi options include self-guided digital programs, brief behavioral treatment programs, and provision of CBTi from trained therapists or psychologists.

## INTRODUCTION

Insomnia and obstructive sleep apnea (OSA) are the two most common sleep disorders and frequently co-occur.[1] The co-occurrence of insomnia and OSA in the same person was first recognized in 1973; however, comorbid insomnia and sleep apnea (COMISA) has only begun to receive an increased amount of research and clinical attention in the past 10 to 15 years.[2] COMISA results in greater morbidity for patients and more complex diagnostic and treatment decisions for clinicians compared with either insomnia or OSA alone.[2] There is evidence that adjunct assessment and management of comorbid insomnia in people with OSA can contribute to improved sleep,

[a] Adelaide Institute for Sleep Health, FHMRI Sleep Health, College of Medicine and Public Health, Flinders University, Bedford Park 5042, Australia; [b] Adelaide Institute for Sleep Health, FHMRI Sleep Health, College of Education, Psychology and Social Work, Flinders University, Bedford Park 5042, Australia; [c] School of Psychological Sciences and Health, University of Strathclyde, Glasgow, United Kingdom; [d] Department of Neurology, Sleep Medicine Division, University of Miami Miller School of Medicine, Miami, FL, USA; [e] Neurology Service, Bruce W. Carter Department of Veterans Affairs Medical Center, Miami, FL, USA
* Corresponding author. Adelaide Institute for Sleep Health, Box 6, Mark Oliphant Building, Level 2A, 5 Laffer Drive, Bedford Park, South Australia 5042, Australia.
E-mail address: alexander.sweetman@flinders.edu.au

Sleep Med Clin 17 (2022) 597–617
https://doi.org/10.1016/j.jsmc.2022.07.006
1556-407X/22/© 2022 Elsevier Inc. All rights reserved.

mental health quality of life, and adherence to OSA therapy. Therefore, it is important to identify and manage comorbid insomnia symptoms among patients with OSA in sleep clinic settings.

OSA is characterized by frequent collapse (apnea) and narrowing (hypopnea) of the upper airway during sleep that results in reduced oxygen saturation, changes in sympathetic activity, and cortical arousals from sleep. This commonly results in fragmented sleep architecture, frequent nocturnal awakenings, and daytime sleepiness and fatigue. OSA results from a combination of anatomical traits (eg, reduced upper airway size) and nonanatomical traits (low respiratory arousal threshold, poor upper airway muscle response, and loop-gain).[3,4] The most common index of OSA presence and severity is the apnea-hypopnea index (AHI), which represents the average number of apneas and hypopneas per hour of sleep. Approximately 10% to 20% of the general population have moderate OSA (AHI $\geq$ 15), although prevalence rates may be much higher.[5-7] OSA results in substantial societal costs through health care use, reduced quality of life, and reduced workplace productivity.[8,9]

Insomnia is characterized by frequent self-reported nocturnal symptoms and associated daytime impairments.[10] Nocturnal symptoms include difficulties initiating sleep, maintaining sleep, and/or undesired early morning awakenings, whereas common daytime symptoms include feelings of fatigue, concentration difficulties, lethargy, poor mood, difficulties with workplace productivity, and increased effort to perform daytime activities.[11] Insomnia may be characterized as an acute (<3 months) or chronic condition ($\geq$3 months). Chronic insomnia occurs in approximately 6% to 15% of adults,[12,13] and is associated with reduced mental health,[14,15] and high societal costs through health care use, reduced productivity, and impaired quality of life.[16] Insomnia frequently co-occurs with other sleep, mental, and physical health problems.[15] When co-occurring with other conditions, insomnia symptoms should be conceptualized as a functionally independent "comorbid" condition, rather than a "secondary symptom."[17] This is because comorbid insomnia often shares bi-directional relationships with other disorders,[18] responds to targeted insomnia treatment,[19] can undermine the management of the comorbid condition if untreated (eg, depression,[20] sleep apnea[1]), and because treatment of the insomnia can also improve management of the comorbid condition.[21,22] As discussed below, this also applies to the management of comorbid insomnia in the presence of OSA.

## COMORBID INSOMNIA AND SLEEP APNEA
### Prevalence of Comorbid Insomnia and Sleep Apnea

The prevalence of COMISA has been investigated in different settings including sleep clinics specializing in the management of OSA, specialist insomnia clinics, primary care settings, military and veteran populations, and in the general population.[1,23,24] It is difficult to estimate the precise prevalence of COMISA, which differs depending on the setting, sampling methods, measures, and specific criteria applied to define each condition.[25] Importantly, the prevalence of COMISA also differs considerably, according to which condition is defined as the "denominator"[26] (Eg, the prevalence of comorbid OSA in patients with insomnia, the prevalence of comorbid insomnia in patients with OSA, or the prevalence of COMISA in the general population). Approximately 30% to 40% of people with insomnia have comorbid OSA, and 30% to 50% of people with OSA report comorbid insomnia symptoms[18] (Fig. 1). Most studies investigating the comorbidity of insomnia and OSA in population-based samples have also reported that insomnia and OSA frequently co-occur.[24,26]

### Characteristics

Compared with people with insomnia alone or OSA alone, those with COMISA experience worse self-reported and objective sleep,[27-29] daytime function,[27,29] mental health,[30,31] and quality of life.[26,32] There is evidence that COMISA is also potentially associated with increased risk of cardio-vascular disease and all-cause mortality in population-based samples.[33-35] A recent study by Lechat and colleagues[36] used the Sleep Heart Health Study to investigate the association of COMISA, insomnia alone, OSA alone, and neither insomnia nor COMISA on risk of all-cause mortality. Participants with COMISA had an increased risk of all-cause mortality (hazard ratio [HR] = 1.47, confidence interval [CI] = 1.06, 2.07) over 15 years of follow-up, compared with participants with neither insomnia/OSA. Insomnia alone and OSA alone were not associated with increased mortality risk. In a sample of 6,877 adults, Sweetman and colleagues also recently reported increased mortality risk in people with self-reported symptoms of COMISA, compared to people with neither condition after adjustment for co-variates (HR = 1.56, CI = 1.06, 2.30).[131] It is possible that the higher morbidity observed in people with COMISA may result from additive effects of the two overlapping sleep disorders, additional comorbidities that may increase the risk of COMISA and morbidity, or interactive effects

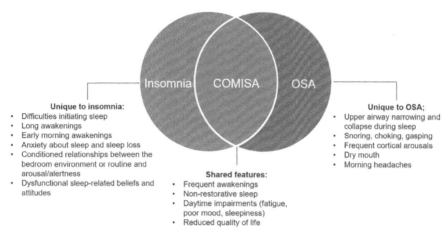

Fig. 1. Comorbid insomnia and sleep apnea (COMISA) is a prevalent condition. Approximately 30% to 50% of people with sleep apnea report insomnia symptoms and 30% to 40% of people with insomnia have comorbid sleep apnea. Insomnia and sleep apnea are characterized by both independent and shared symptoms that can complicate the assessment of COMISA before and following treatment.

between the mechanisms and manifestations of insomnia and OSA on mental and physical health.[18,37] It is also possible that additional sleep-related circadian factors play an important role in the development of COMISA and associations with physical and mental health.[38] Bi-directional relationships between the underlying mechanisms and surfacing symptoms of insomnia, OSA and disturbed sleep, and the impact of these inter-relationships on overall health require further research.[18]

### Secondary Versus Comorbid Insomnia

Diagnostic criteria for chronic insomnia indicate that the sleep-wake difficulty should not be better explained by another sleep disorder.[10,39] Insomnia symptoms may be a direct consequence of apnea and hypopnea events among a subsample of patients with untreated OSA.[40] However, among most patients with COMISA, research indicates that the insomnia responds to targeted insomnia treatment,[29,41] and that insomnia symptoms frequently persist following management of the OSA alone.[40,42] Research has also demonstrated that independent treatment of both conditions improves the overall management of patients with COMISA.[1,2,43] Furthermore, it is difficult to determine causal associations between insomnia and OSA according to baseline symptoms alone,[44,45] and there is evidence suggesting that insomnia and OSA share bi-directional relationships.[18] Therefore, insomnia should be conceptualized as a functionally independent "comorbid" condition with OSA to

encourage targeted assessment and management approaches for both conditions.

### Sociodemographic Factors in Comorbid Insomnia and Sleep Apnea

Some sociodemographic groups may be at increased risk for COMISA but may have a varied clinical presentation that subsequently impacts diagnosis and management. For example, sex differences occur in the presentation of COMISA, with women more likely to report insomnia symptoms and men more likely to report witnessed apneas.[46,47] Additionally, the "disturbed sleep" OSA phenotype is more common among women than men with OSA.[48,49] Age is a known risk factor for both OSA and insomnia, and older age appears to be a risk factor for COMISA.[50] In regards to OSA treatment, both age and sex influence adherence to positive airway pressure (PAP) therapy with younger women using PAP less regularly than older men.[51,52] Despite these age and sex differences in OSA clinical presentation, the treatment approaches and outcomes of COMISA therapies have not been evaluated comprehensively in women versus men or in younger versus older individuals.

Race and ethnicity are other important demographic factors to consider in the presentation and treatment of COMISA. In one study, the OSA "disturbed sleep" phenotype had the highest proportion of Blacks relative to the other four OSA subgroups.[48] Blacks may have an increased prevalence of OSA relative to Whites but poorer adherence to both PAP therapy and cognitive behavioral therapy for insomnia (CBTi).[53,54] Blacks, who on average sleep 1 h less than White individuals, may find the sleep restriction component of CBTi particularly difficult, since their prescribed bedtime window (which is calculated based on their total sleep time) would be lower on average.[55] To date, differences in race/ethnicity have received insufficient attention in randomized controlled trials (RCTs) on COMISA. Thus, it is unknown if these could serve as moderators of treatment outcomes or whether treatments should be culturally/linguistically tailored or delivered via alternative pathways (eg, from trusted community members such as community health care workers).

### Assessment of Insomnia Symptoms

Given that insomnia and OSA are both sleep disorders that impact daytime function, they share several overlapping symptoms (see **Fig. 1**). These shared symptoms can complicate the assessment and diagnosis of insomnia in the presence of OSA. For example, both insomnia and OSA result in more frequent nocturnal awakenings from sleep and are each associated with daytime impairments including poor mood, fatigue, and lethargy.[10,56] This "shared symptoms" phenomenon can complicate the assessment of insomnia symptoms before treatment and after treatment (eg, assessing reduction in insomnia following PAP therapy). Although OSA *and* insomnia result in more frequent brief awakenings from sleep, difficulties returning to sleep after awakening may be a unique symptom of insomnia.

In sleep clinic samples, simple self-report tools can be used to assess patients for insomnia symptoms. For example, the Insomnia Severity Index[57] is a 7-item self-report tool that measures the severity of nocturnal and daytime insomnia symptoms. Higher scores indicate greater insomnia severity. The Sleep Condition Indicator[58] is an 8-item self-report questionnaire for insomnia that maps onto DSM-5 diagnostic criteria. Lower scores indicate worse sleep, with a score of 0 to 16 representing probable insomnia. Because both insomnia and OSA result in similar daytime symptoms, it is important to specifically focus on the presence of nocturnal insomnia symptoms, rather than only the "total" insomnia score of the Insomnia Severity Index or Sleep Condition Indictor, in which daytime symptoms of OSA may contribute heavily to the total insomnia scores.[59,60]

One-week self-report sleep diaries are a useful tool in the assessment of insomnia.[61] Patients can use sleep diaries to self-report their sleep and wake times, when getting out of bed each morning for 1 week. Average nightly sleep onset latency, sleep time, time in bed, wake after sleep onset, and sleep efficiency can be calculated at the end of the week. Sleep diaries can be used to provide an indication of the main types (eg, sleep onset insomnia, sleep maintenance insomnia, early morning awakening insomnia), timing (eg, an "early" or "late" timed body clock), and night-to-night variability/regularity of bedtime behaviors and insomnia symptoms.

## MANAGEMENT APPROACHES FOR COMORBID INSOMNIA AND SLEEP APNEA

An overview of management approaches for COMISA is presented in **Box 1**.

### Insomnia Symptoms Reduce Positive Airway Pressure Adherence

Although continuous PAP therapy is the recommended first-line treatment for moderate and severe OSA, many patients find it difficult to use pressurized masks for the duration of sleep.[62] Consequently, PAP therapy is limited by high rates of immediate rejection, and poor nightly use over time.[63] Patients with insomnia, who already have greater difficulties falling asleep at the start of the night, long awakenings throughout the night, and sleep-related anxiety and catastrophizing beliefs, may have greater difficulty accepting and using PAP therapy, compared with OSA patients without insomnia.[1] It is also suggested that mask discomfort, pressure leaks, and mechanical constraints may exacerbate preexisting insomnia symptoms, and reduce PAP adherence.[64] Several case studies and pilot studies have provided important initial qualitative evidence of the impact of comorbid insomnia on acceptance and use of PAP therapy.[65–67]

A large number of studies investigating the association of comorbid insomnia symptoms with PAP acceptance and use are reported in **Tables 1–3**. Variability in study designs, samples, definitions of insomnia, and measures of PAP adherence make it difficult to synthesize this literature into a single "effect size" estimate. Most studies in this area suggest that patients with lower nightly PAP use are more likely to report insomnia symptoms (cross-sectional associations), and that preexisting insomnia symptoms are associated with lower rates of future PAP adherence (longitudinal associations). Consequently, introducing PAP as the "first-line" treatment for COMISA may result in high rates of treatment rejection and suboptimal adherence, thereby leaving both disorders untreated.

- Patients with confirmed/suspected OSA should be screened for insomnia symptoms and patients reporting insomnia should be assessed for high-risk OSA.

- Treatments for both disorders should be made available to patients with COMISA.

- Treatment sequence may be guided by the patient's chief complaint, severity and temporal onset of symptoms, lifestyle and occupation, comorbid conditions, daytime sleepiness (motor-vehicle risk), and preference for treatment.

- Patients with COMISA have worse acceptance and lower average nightly use of PAP compared with patients with OSA-alone. A subsample of patients with COMISA have adequate PAP use, which improves both the insomnia and OSA. Ongoing research aims to identify this subgroup, to improve precision medicine approaches.

- Cognitive behavioral therapy for insomnia (CBTi) is the recommended "first-line" treatment for chronic insomnia. CBTi is an effective treatment in patients with COMISA and may improve PAP use in those with moderate and severe OSA. Although patients with insomnia alone rarely present with excessive daytime sleepiness, patients with COMISA that present with elevated daytime sleepiness should be monitored closely for increases in daytime sleepiness during the first 2 to 3 weeks of "sleep restriction therapy." See **Table 4** for an overview of CBTi components.

- Sedative-hypnotic medicines are the most common approach to manage insomnia. Early evidence indicated that certain sedative-hypnotics exacerbated OSA in some patients. More recent evidence suggests that specific medicines and combination-medicine approaches may be well tolerated in OSA patients with specific underlying phenotypic traits. Research on sedative-hypnotic medicine tolerance and effectiveness in COMSIA is emerging.

- Some non-PAP therapies for OSA (eg, mandibular advancement splints, surgery) may be effective and well tolerated in specific patients with COMISA. Non-PAP therapies can also be limited by reduced adherence and effectiveness in patients with COMISA compared with those with OSA alone, and research to guide precision medicine approaches is needed.

## Improvements in Insomnia After Positive Airway Pressure

Although insomnia symptoms predict reduced adherence to PAP, a subgroup of patients with COMISA have adequate PAP use, and report improvement in insomnia symptoms following PAP therapy.[40,44] We recently reviewed nine studies investigating the effect of PAP therapy on improving insomnia symptoms and found that PAP improves insomnia by 20% to 50% from baseline levels.[18] An additional recent study by Lundetræ and colleagues[44] investigated the effect of insomnia symptoms on PAP use, and the effect of PAP use on improving insomnia symptoms in 442 patients with OSA. It was reported that although insomnia symptoms predicted worse adherence to PAP therapy, the proportion of patients reporting comorbid insomnia decreased from 51% at baseline to 33% at follow-up. Insomnia improvements were larger among PAP-adherent patients.

These data indicate that some COMISA patients may experience insomnia symptoms as a result of untreated OSA. It is currently very difficult to identify this PAP-responsive subgroup using baseline symptoms alone. Some evidence suggests that greater OSA severity may be associated with more insomnia improvement during PAP.[42] However, higher AHI is also predictive of greater insomnia improvement following CBTi in patients with COMISA.[45] More frequent brief awakenings may also be more responsive to PAP treatment compared with sleep onset/late insomnia.[40] As evidence is still emerging, it is important to consider targeted treatments for each condition when a patient presents with COMISA. Decisions about treatment combinations and sequences should be guided by the patient's "chief complaint," treatment preference, severity and onset of symptoms.

## Non-Positive Airway Pressure Therapies in Comorbid Insomnia and Sleep Apnea

A handful of studies have also investigated the effect, and use of non-PAP therapies in patients with COMISA. Improvement of insomnia symptoms have been reported following upper airway surgery,[89] nasal dilator strip therapy,[90] and mandibular advancement splint therapy.[91] However, patients with COMISA may show reduced acceptance, use, and derive less therapeutic benefit from some of these therapies, compared with patients with OSA alone.[92,93]

## Sedative-Hypnotic Medicines

The use of hypnotic agents and combination pharmacotherapy to manage OSA in patients with

**Table 1**
**Association of insomnia symptoms and adherence to positive airway pressure therapy (1997–2013)**

| Study | N, Age (Mean), Sex, BMI (Mean) | Insomnia Measure and Prevalence | PAP Outcome and Effect of Insomnia on PAP Adherence |
|---|---|---|---|
| Weaver et al,[68] 1997 | 32 patients with confirmed OSA, Age = 47, 81% male, BMI = 40. | After 1 mo of PAP, 42% of patients reported difficulties initiating sleep, and 59% of patients reported frequent awakenings. | Patients were divided into "consistent" vs "intermittent" PAP users at 3-mo follow-up. There was no difference in difficulties initiating sleep between patients characterized as "consistent" (38%), vs "inconsistent" (47%) PAP users. The prevelence of frequent awakenings was lower in patients characterized as "consistent" (44%), vs "inconsistent" (80%) PAP users. |
| Smith et al,[69] 2009 | 52 consecutive OSA patients recommended for PAP. | 57% had at least "moderate" difficulties initiating sleep. | Objective PAP use at 12 mo. Average PAP use was lowest in patients with severe/very severe difficulties initiating sleep (2.7 h/night), compared with those with mild/moderate (5.5 h/night), or no difficulties initiating sleep (6 h/night). |
| Nguyen et al,[70] 2010 | 148 OSA patients, Age = 55, 82% male, BMI = 29. | 49% of patients had a ISI score ≥15. | Objective PAP use and "rejection" were assessed at 1 and 6 mo follow-up. No difference in PAP outcomes were observed between patients with high/low ISI. |
| Wickwire et al,[71] 2010 | 232 OSA patients, Age = 54, 56.5% male, BMI = 34. | 16.6% reported difficulties initiating sleep, 23.7% reported difficulties maintaining sleep and 20.6% reported early morning awakening difficulties. | Average nightly PAP use and levels of adequate "adherence" (≥4 h/night on 70% of nights). After controlling for gender and age, difficulties maintaining sleep predicted lower PAP use and rates of PAP "adherence" at follow-up (variable range of follow-up periods). |

*(continued on next page)*

**Table 1**
(*continued*)

| Study | *N*, Age (Mean), Sex, BMI (Mean) | Insomnia Measure and Prevalence | PAP Outcome and Effect of Insomnia on PAP Adherence |
|---|---|---|---|
| Pieh et al,[72] 2012 | 73 OSA patients, Age = 55, 67% male, BMI = 31. | Regensburg Insomnia Scale (10-item questionnaire). | PAP use was assessed over 6 mo of use. Insomnia symptoms at baseline were not associated with PAP "rejection," but were associated with total PAP use over the first 6 mo. |
| Bjornsdottir et al,[40] 2013 | 705 patients with OSA, Age = 55, 80.6% male, BMI = 34. | Basic Nordic Sleep Questionnaire: 68% were classified with at least one insomnia subtype. | PAP use was assessed via objective and self-report data 2 y after PAP commencement. Difficulties initiating sleep and early morning awakening insomnia were associated with PAP discontinuation after 2 y. The proportion of patients with difficulties maintaining sleep reduced after PAP. |
| Salepci et al,[73] 2013 | 248 OSA patients using PAP (with follow-up data). | Self-reported "difficulties initiating sleep" and "sleep disturbances," assessed at follow-up appointments. | Patients were characterized as PAP adherent ($\geq$4 h/night on 70% of nights) or non-adherent. Difficulties initiating sleep and sleep disturbances were more common among non-adherent patients. |
| Wallace et al,[74] 2013 | 65 Hispanic or Latino veterans with OSA that used PAP and completed follow-up visit. | Average ISI score was 15.6, indicating moderate clinical insomnia. | At 1-wk follow-up, there was no significant difference in ISI scores between PAP adherent vs non-adherent groups. At 1-mo follow-up, the non-adherent group had significantly higher baseline ISI scores ($M = 17, sd = 7$) compared with the adherent group ($M = 13, sd = 5$). |

*Abbreviations:* BMI, body mass index; ISI, insomnia severity index; OSA, obstructive sleep apnea; PAP, positive airway pressure.

**Table 2**
**Association of insomnia symptoms and adherence to positive airway pressure therapy (2014–2017)**

| Study | N, Age (Mean), Sex, BMI (Mean) | Insomnia Measure and Prevalence | PAP Outcome and Effect of Insomnia on PAP Adherence |
|---|---|---|---|
| Glidewell et al,[42] 2014 | 68 OSA patients, Age = 48, 68% male, BMI = 32. | The first 3 items of the ISI were used to define insomnia. 78% of patients had insomnia (ISI subscore ≥4) and 22% had no insomnia. | Objective average nightly PAP use was measured over 1–2 mo. There was no difference in average nightly PAP use between patients with and without insomnia. |
| Stepnowsky et al,[75] 2014 | 241 OSA patients prescribed PAP, Age = 52, 66% male, BMI = 32. | The Pittsburgh Sleep Quality Index was completed after 2 and 4 mo of PAP use. | PAP adherence was negatively associated with Sleep Quality scores at both 2 and 4-mo follow-up. The association of baseline sleep quality with subsequent PAP adherence was not reported. |
| Mysliwiec et al,[76] 2015 | 58 male military personnel with OSA treated with PAP. Age = 36, BMI = 31. | Insomnia (ICSD-3 criteria) classified in 64% of participants. | There was no difference in rates of insomnia, between participants that were adherent (61% insomnia), vs non-adherent (66% insomnia) at 4–6 wk follow-up. |
| Wohlgemuth et al,[77] 2015 | 207 OSA patients, Veterans, Age = 58, 94% male, BMI = 32. | Cross-sectional associations of ISI and PAP adherence were investigated at follow-up. | PAP data were used to identify three subgroups; Non-adherers, Attempters, Adherers. Insomnia severity was higher in PAP "Non-adherers" ($M$ = 15.7) than "Adherers" ($M$ = 8.9). |
| Eysteinsdottir et al,[78] 2016 | 796 OSA patients recommended PAP, Age = 54, 81% male, BMI = 33. | Difficulties initiating sleep, maintaining sleep, and early morning awakenings on the Basic Nordic Sleep Questionnaire. | PAP rejection within 1-y and objective PAP use over past month were investigated. Difficulties initiating sleep and early morning awakening insomnia were associated with PAP rejection. This effect was present in those with BMI≤30, but not those with BMI >30. |

(continued on next page)

**Table 2**
**(continued)**

| Study | N, Age (Mean), Sex, BMI (Mean) | Insomnia Measure and Prevalence | PAP Outcome and Effect of Insomnia on PAP Adherence |
|---|---|---|---|
| Gagnadoux et al,[79] 2016 | 3090 OSA patients with PAP follow-up data | Cluster analysis identified 5 clusters of OSA patients. Clusters 1, 4 had more insomnia symptoms. | PAP "success" (defined as ≥4h use and improved sleepiness/ overall health) was lower in clusters 1, 4, and 5 (representing "female OSA", "mildly symptomatic OSA", and "comorbid OSA" respectively). |
| Saaresranta et al,[49] 2016 | Cluster analysis of patients with OSA (n = 6555). 1067 had PAP data. | Physician diagnosed insomnia, subjective sleep latency ≥30 min, self-reported sleep duration ≤6 h and/or use of hypnotics. | Divided participants into four groups depending on presence vs absence of insomnia and excessive daytime sleepiness. Trends for lower PAP adherence in groups with insomnia, and higher PAP adherence in group with sleepiness but no insomnia, after controlling for age, BMI and gender. |
| Lam et al,[64] 2017 | 172 patients (123 with ISI data) presenting to a clinic for "PAP-intolerant patients." | ISI was completed before treatment. | Of patients with available ISI data, 59% had at least moderate insomnia. The most frequent reasons for PAP rejection/failure were; claustrophobia, mask discomfort, and sleeping difficulty. |
| Libman et al,[80] 2017 | 29 female OSA patients, Age = 65, BMI = 32. | ISI, Sleep questionnaire (nightly awakenings, fatigue, sleepiness, sleep quality). | Self-reported PAP use was collected after 2 y. Participants were defined as "adherent" vs "non-adherent" (≥4h use on ≥80% of nights). The ISI did not predict PAP adherence group. |

*Abbreviations:* BMI, body mass index; ISI, insomnia severity index; OSA, obstructive sleep apnea; PAP, positive airway pressure.

specific phenotypes is an exciting emerging area.[94] Sedative-hypnotic medicines including benzodiazepines and "z-drugs" are a common approach to manage insomnia.[95,96] However, they are not recommended as "first-line" treatment or a long-term management approach for insomnia, due to potential for dependence, side-effects, and tolerance to therapeutic dose.[97–99]

Hypnotic medicines may be well tolerated and improve sleep in specific OSA patients.[94] For example, a low respiratory arousal threshold is one of the main nonanatomical contributors to

**Table 3**
**Association of insomnia symptoms and adherence to positive airway pressure therapy (2018 – current)**

| Study | N, Age (Mean), Sex, BMI (Mean) | Insomnia Measure and Prevalence | PAP Outcome and Effect of Insomnia on PAP Adherence |
|---|---|---|---|
| Cho et al,[81] 2018 | 77 of 476 prospectively screened OSA patients with PAP follow-up data. Age = 51, 76% male, BMI = 26. | ISI ≥15 was used to identify patients with insomnia (29%). Cross-sectional associations with PAP adherence were investigated. | Among the 77 patients with PAP data, there was no difference in adherence to PAP therapy between OSA patients with and without insomnia. There was no correlation between the ISI and PAP adherence. |
| El-Solh et al,[82] 2018 | 72 Veterans with OSA and Post-Traumatic Stress Disorder. Age = 50, 79% male, BMI = 34. | ISI ≥15 was used to identify patients with insomnia at baseline (50%). | Participants with COMISA used PAP for fewer nights (33%) than those without insomnia (50%) at 12-wk follow-up. |
| Philip et al,[83] 2018 | 288 OSA patients. Age = 63, 69% male, BMI = 30. | Cross-sectional assessment of PAP adherence with insomnia (ISI), self-efficacy and other self-report data. | PAP adherence was negatively correlated with the ISI total score, and nocturnal insomnia item score; difficulties initiating sleep, and difficulties maintaining sleep. |
| Fichten et al,[84] 2018 (abstract) | 46 OSA patients prescribed PAP. Age = 54. | Self-reported difficulties initiating and maintaining sleep, and insomnia was assessed before and 1.5 y after PAP therapy. | 20 of 46 participants were categorized as PAP-adherent at follow-up. Insomnia symptoms were less prevalent in the PAP adherent (20% had insomnia) than the non-adherent group (38% had insomnia). |
| Park et al,[85] 2018 | 359 OSA patients. Age = 58, 78% male, BMI = 26. | The total ISI score, and itemized responses were investigated. | PAP adherence (defined as the use of PAP for ≥4 h per night on 70% of nights) was observed in 46% of participants. Sleep onset insomnia symptoms (but not overall insomnia severity) were associated with PAP non-adherence. |

(continued on next page)

**Table 3**
**(continued)**

| Study | N, Age (Mean), Sex, BMI (Mean) | Insomnia Measure and Prevalence | PAP Outcome and Effect of Insomnia on PAP Adherence |
|---|---|---|---|
| Sawunyavisuth,[86] 2018 | 53 OSA patients recommended PAP therapy, Age = 56, 62% male, BMI = 30. | Questionnaire assessing side effects resulting from trial of PAP. Included insomnia symptoms. | Following PAP trial, 12 patients (23%) did not purchase PAP and 41 patients (77%) did purchase PAP. Patients that did not purchase PAP indicated more insomnia symptoms, tightness of mask, cough and irritation resulting from PAP trial. |
| Wallace et al,[87] 2018 | 53 Veterans with OSA that initiated PAP. Age = 50, 96% male, BMI = 34. | A ISI subscore $\geq 6$ (three nocturnal items) was used to identify patients with insomnia (47%). | At 6-mo follow-up, participants with comorbid insomnia had significantly lower average PAP use (2.8 h) compared with participants without comorbid insomnia (4 h/night). Participants with comorbid insomnia also had a lower percentage of days with at least 4 h use (32%), vs to those without comorbid insomnia (50%). |
| Drakou et al,[88] 2021 | 272 patients with suspected OSA, Age = 53, 74% male, BMI = 34. 160 recommended PAP. | Athens Insomnia Scale score $\geq 10$. | Among patients with severe OSA and mild depression, those with insomnia were less likely to initially accept PAP therapy (25%) compared with those with no comorbid insomnia (59%). There was no effect of insomnia presence on acceptance of PAP in patients with moderate OSA, or those without depression symptoms. |

*Abbreviations:* BMI, body mass index; ISI, insomnia severity index; OSA, obstructive sleep apnea; PAP, positive airway pressure.

OSA pathogenesis.[4] At least one-third of OSA patients have a low respiratory arousal threshold, in which they awaken to increasing respiratory effort and relatively minor airway narrowing, thereby perpetuating breathing instability.[18,100] Consequently, it is thought that increasing the arousal threshold may be a therapeutic target to improve overall airway stability in such patients. Ongoing research aims to investigate the low arousal threshold as a common mechanistic feature of OSA and COMISA.[18] Several studies have investigated the effect of different hypnotic/combination agents in patients with OSA.[101] Messineo and colleagues[102] recently reported that zolpidem (10 mg) results in an increase in objective sleep efficiency and respiratory arousal threshold, but no change in AHI, versus placebo, in patients with OSA and a low-to-moderate arousal threshold. A recent RCT by Cheng and colleagues[103] also investigated the effect of 10 mg Lemborexant (a dual orexin receptor antagonist) in patients with mild OSA. It was reported that Lemborexant did not increase AHI, or reduce mean oxygen saturation, or percentage of sleep time with oxygen saturation less than 90%, versus placebo.

There is a growing trend in off-label antidepressant and antipsychotic medicines prescribed to manage insomnia.[15,104] Most studies investigating the effect of antidepressants for insomnia have been limited to small samples and short-term follow-up.[105] Consequently, these medicines are not presently recommended for the management of insomnia.[15] Antipsychotic medicines may also lead to a substantial AHI increase in patients presenting with insomnia symptoms.[106] Based on this limited evidence and potential for exacerbation of OSA, antidepressant and antipsychotic medicines are not currently recommended for the management of insomnia or COMISA.

### Cognitive Behavioral Therapy for Insomnia is the Most Effective Treatment for Insomnia

CBTi is the recommended "first-line" treatment for chronic insomnia.[99,107,108] CBTi is a multicomponent therapy that aims to identify and gradually reduce the underlying psychological, behavioral and physiologic factors that maintain the insomnia condition.[109] CBTi includes several therapeutic components that may be tailored to patients' presenting symptoms and underlying features of the disorder (**Table 4**). Because CBTi targets the underlying causes of insomnia, it leads to improvements in sleep, daytime function, and mental health that are sustained long after therapy cessation. CBTi is commonly administered by trained therapists/psychologists over 6 to 8 weekly/fortnightly sessions, but has also been translated to self-guided reading, audio, and interactive online programs. A brief behavioral therapy for insomnia has been developed,[110,111] which distils the most effective educational and behavioral treatment components (stimulus control therapy, and bedtime restriction therapy) into a succinct 4-session program that can be delivered in a diverse range of health care settings.[112] As many patients with COMISA spend at least 4 weeks between their PAP titration and setup/initiation appointments, brief CBTi programs could

be delivered without delaying commencement of PAP therapy.

CBTi is an effective and safe treatment in the presence of untreated OSA.[29,41,113] Several case studies, pilot studies, and four recent RCTs (**Table 5**) have investigated the effect of CBTi on acceptance and use of PAP therapy. Evidence suggests that face-to-face CBTi interventions improve insomnia in the presence of OSA, can be safely delivered before OSA treatment, and may increase subsequent acceptance and use of PAP therapy in those with moderate and severe OSA.[114–117] Mixed results in this area (see **Table 5**) highlight the need for further research to identify the most effective treatment sequence/s, interventions, and specific COMISA patients that are most responsive to CBTi before commencing PAP. There is also RCT evidence that CBTi reduces OSA severity through sleep consolidation.[22]

Adherence to CBTi in COMISA patients has not been evaluated yet, but there are specific issues that need attention, especially when CBTi and PAP therapy are provided simultaneously. For example, a patient with sleep onset insomnia symptoms might struggle to adhere to stimulus control instructions to get out of bed if unable to sleep (see **Table 4**), as this would require removal and replacement of PAP equipment on each occasion. If stimulus control therapy is indicated as the best treatment for the insomnia, it could be initiated a couple of weeks before PAP commencement by which time repeated times out of bed should no longer be necessary. Another consideration for combined treatment is that some patients (particularly those including long reported periods awake in bed) being administered bedtime restriction therapy, will be asked to restrict their time in bed, in some cases as low as 5.5 hrs. This needs to be communicated to the care provider evaluating PAP adherence, who needs to acknowledge that PAP use will not be beyond those 5.5 h (assuming the patient is adherent to their prescribed time in bed). A move away from "PAP adherence based on hours of use" toward "PAP adherence based on % of time in bed with effective therapy" may be considered. This metric would be similar to psychologists using "sleep efficiency" rather than "total sleep time" to assess treatment-response to CBTi.

### Increasing access to cognitive behavioral therapy for insomnia in sleep clinics

Despite strong recommendations that CBTi should be used as the "first-line" treatment for insomnia,[98,107,108] and evidence that CBTi is effective and safe[118] in the presence of comorbid OSA, most clinicians and patients lack access to CBTi.

**Table 4**
**Components of cognitive behavioral therapy for insomnia (CBTi)**

| Component | Description |
|---|---|
| Education about sleep | CBTi programs commonly begin with information about the process that control our sleep (2-process model).<br>Sleep hygiene information is not an adequate stand-alone treatment for insomnia, but can be helpful in providing a treatment rationale for other active treatment components.<br>Sleep information can also be used to provide accurate information about some of the common myths and misconceptions about sleep (see Cognitive Therapy below). |
| Stimulus control therapy | Instructions to help patients fall asleep quicker at the start of the night and following nocturnal awakenings;<br>1. Use the bed only for sleep and intimacy,<br>2. Get up at the same time each morning,<br>3. Only go to bed when sleepy, do not "try hard" to fall asleep,<br>4. If not asleep within approximately 15-min, get out of bed and go to another room until sleepy again,<br>5. Repeat steps 3 and 4 until asleep,<br>6. Repeat steps 3 and 4 in the middle of the night when awake,<br>7. Avoid daytime naps (especially long naps). |
| Bedtime restriction therapy (also called *sleep restriction therapy*) | Aims to reduce the "conditioned" relationship between being in bed with a state of alertness and arousal. Patients are guided to temporarily reduce the time they spend in bed over multiple consecutive nights. This may result in a small amount of sleep loss during the first 1–2 wk. Sleep pressure will increase during the first 1–2 wk of therapy. This promotes quicker sleep onset and reduces the length of nocturnal awakenings. As patients begin sleeping for the large majority of time they spend in bed (85%), their time in bed can gradually be extended from week-to-week until a comfortable and satisfying equilibrium between their sleep efficiency (% of time in bed asleep), and daytime sleepiness is achieved. Typically, the prescribed time in bed is never reduced below 5.5 h. |
| Cognitive therapy | Aims to identify and challenge the patient's maladaptive beliefs about sleep. These beliefs are replaced with more realistic ones that help the patient adopt a more accurate understanding of the impact of poor sleep on daytime functioning, sleep needs, and sleep medication. Techniques such as Socratic questioning or behavioral experiments are often part of cognitive therapy. |
| Relaxation therapy | Includes progressive muscle relaxation, mindfulness therapies, and meditation that aims to reduce alertness and arousal before bed and throughout the night. Relaxation exercises should be practiced over multiple days/nights to improve this cognitive skill, rather than as a once-off treatment. |

This clear deficiency of CBTi requires attention. This may be achieved through embedding psychologists with training in CBTi in sleep clinics that specialize in OSA, or developing referral networks between sleep clinics and external "sleep" psychologists. Secondly, CBTi programs have been translated to a brief behavioral therapy,[111] that may be delivered by existing PAP nurses, or other clinicians in sleep clinic settings. It may also be possible to up-skill family physicians, community health care professionals and social workers to administer this brief behavioral treatment for insomnia to improve availability.[112] CBTi may be delivered via telemedicine to increase access in rural/remote and underserved areas.[119] Finally, CBTi programs have also been translated to self-guided digital programs.[120] Digital CBTi is an effective treatment for insomnia that also improves comorbid depression and anxiety symptoms.[121,122] At least one ongoing study is evaluating the effect of digital CBTi in patients with COMISA.[113] This research may inform

**Table 5**
**Randomized controlled trials investigating effect of CBTi on insomnia symptoms and PAP adherence in patients with COMISA**

| Study | Sample Characteristics | Design | Insomnia Outcome | OSA Outcome |
|---|---|---|---|---|
| Bjorvatn et al,[117] 2018 | 164 patients with COMISA (Age M = 56, 71% male, BMI M = 32). | Parallel-arm RCT of a self-help book vs sleep hygiene concurrent with PAP therapy, on insomnia symptoms and PAP adherence. | There was no between-group difference in change in insomnia symptoms from pretreatment to 3-mo follow-up. | There was no between-group difference in PAP adherence. |
| Sweetman et al,[114] 2019 | 145 patients with COMISA (Age M = 59, 56% male, BMI M = 35). | Parallel-arm RCT of CBTi, vs no-treatment, on insomnia symptoms, and PAP acceptance/adherence in patients with untreated COMISA. | CBTi group experienced greater reduction in insomnia severity by post-CBTi/control, and 6-mo follow-up, vs control. | CBTi group had greater initial acceptance (99 vs 89%) and long term nightly use of PAP, vs control (61 min difference). |
| Ong et al,[115] 2020 | 121 patients with COMISA (Age M = 50, 55% male). | 3-arm RCT of CBTi before PAP, CBTi concurrent with PAP, and PAP-only on insomnia symptoms and PAP adherence in 121 PAP naïve COMISA patients. | Compared with patients receiving PAP only, those receiving combined CBTi and PAP experienced greater improvement of the ISI. There was no difference between the groups that received sequential CBTi before PAP, vs concurrent CBTi and PAP. | There were no significant between-group differences in PAP adherence. |
| Alessi et al,[116] 2021 | 124 veterans with COMISA (Age M = 63, 96% male). | Parallel-arm RCT of integrated CBTi + PAP adherence intervention, vs no-treatment, on insomnia symptoms and PAP adherence in veterans with COMISA. | Compared with the control group, the CBTi group experienced greater improvement in the ISI, self-report, and actigraphy measures sleep parameters. | Compared with the control group, the CBTi group had greater average nightly PAP use at 3 mo (3.0, vs 1.9 h/night) and 6-mo follow-up (2.4, vs 1.5 h/night). |

Abbreviations: CBTi, cognitive behavioral therapy for insomnia; ISI, insomnia severity index; PAP, positive airway pressure; RCT, randomized controlled trial.
Adapted from Sweetman et al., (2019).[2]

the feasibility of a stepped-care system for management of insomnia in patients with COMISA.

## Proposed mechanisms

The pathophysiology and developmental course of COMISA remains unclear and the exact mechanisms remain somewhat elusive because of the lack of research in this area. Understanding the mechanisms underpinning COMISA is important, as this will likely improve precision medicine approaches for future patients, and potentially highlight areas for early intervention to prevent development and/or exacerbation of COMISA.[18] It is likely that there are multiple pathways that lead to the development of COMISA, so only a handful of mechanisms are discussed below.

**Effect of obstructive sleep apnea on insomnia** The most common proposed pathway is that OSA is a precipitating factor for insomnia, increasing the risk of the development of chronic insomnia.[18] Specifically, arousals due to respiratory events result in sleep disruptions and increased sympathetic activity. Over time, the nocturnal increase in sympathetic activity associated with these respiratory events and awakenings could lead to periods of wakefulness, (mis)perceptions of multiple brief sleep periods as continued wakefulness,[123] feelings of frustration and anxiety about sleep loss, maladaptive behaviors and a state of chronic hyperarousal, one of the hallmark symptoms of insomnia disorder.[124] Over time, the insomnia condition may develop functional independence of the OSA, or remain partly dependent on respiratory-induced arousals/awakenings in some patients with COMISA.

Another possible mechanism is through rapid eye movement (REM) instability. Respiratory events disproportionally occur during REM sleep and light sleep in patients with OSA.[125] Respiratory events during REM sleep may lead to more frequent arousals and disruption of REM sleep. Riemann and colleagues proposed that such instability of REM sleep and frequent arousals might offer an explanation for the development of sleep maintenance insomnia, as these arousals contribute to the misperception of vivid dream mentation as wakefulness.[126] Although this proposed pathway does not explain the development of sleep onset insomnia symptoms, it is supported by research indicating that nocturnal awakenings in insomnia patients are often triggered by respiratory events.[127] This conceptualization is somewhat intuitive and consistent with the outdated conceptualization that insomnia is often secondary to co-occurring physical and mental health conditions (ie, "secondary insomnia"). However,

as outlined above, PAP is not necessarily the most advantageous "first-line" treatment for all COMISA patients, especially those with sleep onset difficulties, or nocturnal awakenings and difficulties returning to sleep.

**Effect of insomnia on obstructive sleep apnea** A second, albeit less intuitive pathway, is that insomnia disorder leads to the exacerbation of OSA in patients with a pre-existing anatomic predisposition. It has been suggested that partial sleep deprivation experienced during periods of insomnia may compromise upper airway muscle tone.[128,129] The effect of sleep deprivation (including multiple nights of partial sleep restriction) on OSA severity and upper airway muscle tone in the context of insomnia and COMISA requires further research.[18] Alternatively, insomnia disorder that is characterized by a state of increased cognitive and physiologic arousal during the day and night (hyper-arousal), may contribute to a reduced respiratory arousal threshold, one of the main nonanatomical traits of OSA.[4] A recent study showed a small reduction of the AHI in COMISA patients following treatment of insomnia with CBTi.[22] The authors speculate that consolidating periods of fragmented sleep might improve airway patency, or that the increased homeostatic drive for sleep seen with sleep restriction therapy may lead to an increase in the respiratory arousal threshold. This preliminary data certainly supports the notion of providing CBTi before the initiation of PAP therapy.

**Common underlying pathophysiology** Benetó and colleagues[130] speculate that the hypothalamic–pituitary–adrenal (HPA) axis might play an important role in the development of COMISA. The authors hypothesize a reciprocal relationship between OSA and insomnia mediated by activation of the HPA axis, which is caused by sleep fragmentation, reduced sleep duration and chronic sleep deprivation common to both conditions. The authors acknowledge an established evidence base for the effect of OSA on HPA axis activation, but that most of the research on insomnia has focused on the HPA axis activation as a cause for insomnia. Much less clear is the potential of HPA axis activation as a consequence of insomnia and cause for OSA, which would support their hypothesis of the HPA axis activation as the common link and mediator of the reciprocal relationship between OSA and insomnia. Research that links HPA activation and insomnia with objective short sleep duration supports the hypothesis that within this subgroup, HPA axis activation may be a consequence of insomnia. Additionally, metabolic syndrome has been proposed as a cause for OSA; metabolic syndrome in turn is a direct consequence of increased HPA axis activation. Together these results support the hypothesis that HPA axis activation may be a cause and consequence of each disorder, leading to a reciprocal relationship between insomnia and OSA.

It is likely that multiple pathways contribute to the development of COMISA. More longitudinal and experimental studies are needed to test possible mechanisms between insomnia and OSA. Certainly, information about these mechanisms will help guide our treatment approaches.

## SUMMARY

Insomnia and sleep apnea are the two most common sleep disorders and frequently co-occur. COMISA results in greater morbidity for patients, and complex diagnostic and treatment decisions for clinicians. It is important for sleep clinicians to assess for insomnia symptoms among patients with suspected/confirmed OSA, and provide access to treatments for both disorders. CBTi is an effective insomnia treatment in the presence of untreated OSA, and may improve adherence to PAP therapy in patients with moderate/severe OSA. Many sleep clinics worldwide currently specialize in the diagnosis and management of OSA alone, and should consider incorporating insomnia and COMISA management pathways to improve outcomes for patients with COMISA.

## CLINICS CARE POINTS

- Comorbid insomnia and sleep apnea (COMISA) frequently co-occur. This results in worse sleep, daytime function, and quality of life, compared with either disorder alone.

- It is important to implement evidence-based insomnia assessment and management approaches in sleep clinics worldwide to improve the management of COMISA.

- Clinicians may screen for insomnia symptoms in patients with suspected and confirmed obstructive sleep apnea (OSA). Clinicians should be aware of the shared and unique symptoms of each disorder than can complicate the assessment and diagnostic process in patients with COMISA (see **Fig. 1**).

- Patients with COMISA should be offered treatments for both disorders.

- Patients with COMISA have lower nightly use of positive airway pressure (PAP) therapy,

compared with patients with OSA alone (**Tables 1–3**).

- A subsample of patients with COMISA shows adequate use of PAP therapy that improves symptoms of insomnia and OSA. There is currently insufficient evidence to identify this PAP-responsive group of COMISA patients before commencing treatment (ie, precision medicine approaches). This is an important area of emerging research.

- Cognitive behavioral therapy for insomnia (CBTi; see **Table 4**) is the most effective and recommended "first-line" treatment for (comorbid) insomnia. CBTi is effective and safe in the presence of mild, moderate, and severe OSA. Patients should be monitored for increased daytime sleepiness during the first 1 to 2 weeks of "bedtime restriction therapy" (one of the core therapeutic components of CBTi).

- There is evidence that CBTi improves acceptance and use of PAP therapy among patients with comorbid insomnia and moderate and severe OSA (see **Table 5**).

## DISCLOSURE

D.M. Wallace has no conflicts of interest to declare. A. Sweetman and L. Lack declare research funding and equipment support from the National Health and Medical Research Council (NHMRC), Flinders Foundation, ResMed, and Philips Respironics. A. Sweetman is supported by an NHMRC Centres of Research Excellence grant (GNT1134954). L. Lack has received research funding and is a shareholder of Re-time Aus. M. Crawford has received research funding from Brain Research UK and Chief Scientist Office.

## REFERENCES

1. Sweetman A, Lack L, Catcheside P, et al. Developing a successful treatment for comorbid insomnia and sleep apnoea. Sleep Med Rev 2017;33:28–38.
2. Sweetman A, Lack L, Bastien C. Comorbid insomnia and sleep apnea (COMISA): prevalence, consequences, methodological considerations, and recent randomized controlled trials. Brain Sci 2019;9(12):371.
3. Eckert DJ. Phenotypic approaches to obstructive sleep apnoea–new pathways for targeted therapy. Sleep Med Rev 2018;37:45–59.
4. Osman AM, Carter SG, Carberry JC, et al. Obstructive sleep apnea: current perspectives. Nat Sci Sleep 2018;10:21.

5. Peppard PE, Young T, Barnet JH, et al. Increased prevalence of sleep-disordered breathing in adults. Am J Epidemiol 2013;177(9):1006–14.

6. Heinzer R, Vat S, Marques-Vidal P, et al. Prevalence of sleep-disordered breathing in the general population: the HypnoLaus study. Lancet Respir Med 2015;3(4):310–8.

7. Benjafield AV, Ayas NT, Eastwood PR, et al. Estimation of the global prevalence and burden of obstructive sleep apnoea: a literature-based analysis. Lancet Respir Med 2019;7(8):687–98.

8. Deloitte Access Economics, Re-awakening Australia: The economic cost of sleep disorders in Australia. Sydney, Australia2010.

9. AlGhanim N, Comondore VR, Fleetham J, et al. The economic impact of obstructive sleep apnea. Lung 2008;186:7–12.

10. The American Academy of Sleep Medicine. 3rd ed. International Classification of Sleep Disorders (ICSD-3), Diagnostic and coding manual: Westchester, IL; 2014.

11. Bickley K, Lovato N, Lack L. The sleep impact on activity diary (SIAD): a novel assessment of daytime functioning in insomnia. Brain Sci 2021;11(2):219.

12. Ohayon M. Epidemiology of insomnia: what we know and what we still need to learn. Sleep Med Rev 2002;6(2):97–111.

13. Reynolds A, Appleton S, Gill T, Adams R. Chronic insomnia disorder in Australia: A report to the Sleep Health Foundation. Sleep Health Foundation Special Report. 2019.

14. Baglioni C, Battagliese G, Feige B, et al. Insomnia as a predictor of depression: a meta-analytic evaluation of longitudinal epidemiological studies. J Affect Disord 2011;135(1–3):10–9.

15. Sweetman A, Van Ryswyk E, Vakulin A, et al. Co-occurring depression and insomnia in Australian primary care: a narrative review of recent scientific evidence. Med J Aust 2021;215(5):230–6.

16. Natsky A, Vakulin A, Chai-Coetzer C, et al. Economic evaluation of cognitive behavioural therapy for insomnia (CBT-I) for improving health outcomes in adult populations: a systematic review. Sleep Med Rev 2020;54:101351.

17. Lichstein KL. Secondary insomnia: a myth dismissed. Sleep Med Rev 2006;10(1):3–5.

18. Sweetman A, Lack L, McEvoy RD, et al. Bi-directional relationships between comorbid insomnia and sleep apnea (COMISA). Sleep Med Rev 2021;101519.

19. Sweetman A, Lovato N, Micic G, et al. Do symptoms of depression, anxiety or stress impair the effectiveness of cognitive behavioral therapy for insomnia? A chart-review of 455 patients with chronic insomnia. Sleep Med 2020;75:401–10.

20. Dombrovski AY, Cyranowski JM, Mulsant BH, et al. Which symptoms predict recurrence of depression in women treated with maintenance interpersonal psychotherapy? Depress Anxiety 2008;25(12):1060–6.

21. Cheng P, Kalmbach DA, Tallent G, et al. Depression prevention via digital cognitive behavioral therapy for insomnia: a randomized controlled trial. Sleep 2019;42(10):zsz150.

22. Sweetman A, Lack L, McEvoy D, et al. Cognitive behavioural therapy for insomnia reduces sleep apnoea severity: a randomised controlled trial. ERJ OR 2020;6(2). 00161-2020.

23. Luyster FS, Buysse DJ, Strollo PJ. Comorbid insomnia and obstructive sleep apnea: challenges for clinical practice and research. J Clin Sleep Med 2010;6(2):196–204.

24. Zhang Y, Ren R, Lei F, et al. Worldwide and regional prevalence rates of co-occurrence of insomnia and insomnia symptoms with obstructive sleep apnea: a systematic review and meta-analysis. Sleep Med Rev 2019;45:1–17.

25. Uhlig B, Hagen K, Engstrøm M, et al. The relationship between obstructive sleep apnea and insomnia: a population-based cross-sectional polysomnographic study 2019;54:126–33.

26. Sweetman A, Melaku YA, Lack L, et al. Prevalence and associations of comorbid insomnia and sleep apnoea (COMISA) in an Australian population-based sample. Sleep Med 2021;82:9–17.

27. Krakow B, Melendrez D, Ferreira E, et al. Prevalence of insomnia symptoms in patients with sleep-disordered breathing. Chest 2001;120(6):1923–9.

28. Bianchi M, Williams KL, McKinney S, et al. The subjective-objective mismatch in sleep perception among those with insomnia and sleep apnea. J Sleep Res 2013;22(5):557–68.

29. Sweetman A, Lack LC, Lambert S, et al. Does co-morbid obstructive sleep apnea impair the effectiveness of cognitive and behavioral therapy for insomnia? Sleep Med 2017;39:38–46.

30. Jeon B, Luyster FS, Callan JA, et al. Depressive symptoms in comorbid obstructive sleep apnea and insomnia: an integrative review. West J Nurs Res 2021. https://doi.org/10.1177/0193945921989656. 0193945921989656.

31. Lang CJ, Appleton SL, Vakulin A, et al. Co-morbid OSA and insomnia increases depression prevalence and severity in men. Respirology 2017;22:1407–15.

32. Tasbakan MS, Gunduz C, Pirildar S, et al. Quality of life in obstructive sleep apnea is related to female gender and comorbid insomnia. Sleep and Breathing 2018;1–8.

33. Meira e Cruz M, Salles C, Gozal D. A Reappraisal on the associations between sleep-disordered breathing, insomnia and Cardiometabolic risk. Am J Respir Crit Care Med 2021;203(12):1583–4.

34. Vozoris NT. Sleep apnea-plus: prevalence, risk factors, and association with cardiovascular diseases using United States population-level data. Sleep Med 2012;13(6):637–44.

35. Lechat B, Appleton S, Melaku Y, et al. Comorbid insomnia and obstructive sleep apnoea is associated with all-cause mortality and cardiovascular event risk. Brisbane, Australia: Sleep Down Under; 2021.

36. Lechat B, Appleton S, Melaku Y, et al. Comorbid insomnia and obstructive sleep apnoea is associated with all-cause mortality. European Respiratory Journal 2021;in press.

37. Meira e Cruz M, Sweetman A. Insomnia, sleep apnea, and circadian misalignment as a "three-arm" contributor to anxiety and depression during pregnancy. Sleep Vigilance 2021;1–3.

38. Sweetman A, Reynolds A, Lack LC. Circadian factors in comorbid insomnia and sleep apnea (COMISA). J Clin Sleep Med 2021;17(9):1959–60.

39. Bjorvatn B, Jernelöv S, Pallesen S. Insomnia–a heterogenic disorder often comorbid with psychological and somatic disorders and diseases: a comprehensive review with focus on diagnostic and treatment challenges. Front Psychol 2021;12:289.

40. Björnsdóttir E, Janson C, Sigurdsson JF, et al. Symptoms of insomnia among patients with obstructive sleep apnea before and after two years of positive airway pressure treatment. Sleep 2013;36(12):1901–9.

41. Fung CH, Martin JL, Josephson K, et al. Efficacy of cognitive behavioral therapy for insomnia in older adults with occult sleep-disordered breathing. Psychosom Med 2016;78(5):629–39.

42. Glidewell RN, Renn BN, Roby E, et al. Predictors and patterns of insomnia symptoms in OSA before and after PAP therapy. Sleep Med 2014;15(8):899–905.

43. Ong JC, Crawford MR, Wallace DM. Sleep apnea and insomnia: emerging evidence for effective clinical management. Chest 2020;159(5):2020–8.

44. Lundetræ RS, Saxvig IW, Aurlien H, et al. Effect of continuous positive airway pressure on symptoms and prevalence of insomnia in patients with obstructive sleep apnea: a longitudinal study. Front Psychol 2021;12:691495.

45. Sweetman A, Lechat B, Catcheside PG, et al. Polysomnographic predictors of treatment response to cognitive behavioral therapy for insomnia in participants with comorbid insomnia and sleep apnea: secondary analysis of a randomized controlled trial. Front Psychol 2021;12:1613.

46. Shepertycky MR, Banno K, Kryger M. Differences between men and women in the clinical presentation of patients diagnosed with obstructive sleep apnea syndrome. Sleep 2005;28(3):309–14.

47. Subramanian S, Guntupalli B, Murugan T, et al. Gender and ethnic differences in prevalence of self-reported insomnia among patients with obstructive sleep apnea. Sleep Breath 2011;15(4):711–5.

48. Keenan BT, Kim J, Singh B, et al. Recognizable clinical subtypes of obstructive sleep apnea across international sleep centers: a cluster analysis. Sleep 2018;41(3):zsx214.

49. Saaresranta T, Hedner J, Bonsignore MR, et al. Clinical phenotypes and comorbidity in European sleep apnoea patients. PloS one 2016;11(10):e0163439.

50. Lichstein KL, Riedel BW, Lester KW, et al. Occult sleep apnea in a recruited sample of older adults with insomnia. J Consult Clin Psychol 1999;67(3):405–10.

51. Woehrle H, Graml A, Weinreich G. Age-and gender-dependent adherence with continuous positive airway pressure therapy. Sleep Med 2011;12(10):1034–6.

52. Patel S, Bakker J, Stitt C, et al. Age and sex disparities in adherence to CPAP. Chest 2021;159(1):382–9.

53. Wallace DM, Williams NJ, Sawyer AM, et al. Adherence to positive airway pressure treatment among minority populations in the US: a scoping review. Sleep Med Rev 2018;38:56–69.

54. El-Solh AA, O'Brien N, Akinnusi M, et al. Predictors of cognitive behavioral therapy outcomes for insomnia in veterans with post-traumatic stress disorder. Sleep Breath 2019;23(2):635–43.

55. Williams N, Jean-Louis G, Blanc J, et al. Race, socioeconomic position and sleep. Sleep Health 2019;57–76.

56. Chervin RD. Sleepiness, fatigue, tiredness, and lack of energy in obstructive sleep apnea. Chest 2000;118(2):372–9.

57. Bastien CH, Vallières A, Morin CM. Validation of the insomnia severity index as an outcome measure for insomnia research. Sleep Med 2001;2(4):297–307.

58. Espie CA, Kyle SD, Hames P, et al. The Sleep Condition Indicator: a clinical screening tool to evaluate insomnia disorder. BMJ open 2014;4(3):e004183.

59. Wallace DM, Wohlgemuth WK. Predictors of insomnia severity index profiles in US veterans with obstructive sleep apnea. J Clin Sleep Med 2019;15(12):1827–37.

60. Sweetman A, Lack L, McEvoy D. Refining the Measurement of Insomnia in Patients with Obstructive Sleep Apnea: Wallace, et al., Predictors of Insomnia Severity Index Profiles in US veterans with Obstructive Sleep Apnea (JC-19-00217). J Clin Sleep Med 2019;15(12):1717–9.

61. Carney CE, Buysse DJ, Ancoli-Israel S, et al. The consensus sleep diary: standardizing prospective sleep self-monitoring. Sleep 2012;35(2):287–302.

62. Weaver TE, Grunstein RR. Adherence to continuous positive airway pressure therapy: the challenge to effective treatment. Proc Am Thorac Soc 2008;5(2):173–8.

63. Epstein LJ, Kristo D, Strollo PJ, et al. Clinical guideline for the evaluation, management and long-term care of obstructive sleep apnea in adults: adult obstructive sleep apnea task force of the American Academy of Sleep Medicine. J Clin Sleep Med 2009;5(3):263–76.

64. Lam AS, Collop NA, Bliwise DL, et al. Validated measures of insomnia, function, sleepiness, and nasal obstruction in a CPAP alternatives clinic population. J Clin Sleep Med 2017;13(8):949–57.

65. Wickwire EM, Schumacher JA, Richert AC, et al. Combined insomnia and poor CPAP compliance: a case study and discussion. Clin Case Stud 2008;7(4):267–86.

66. Suraiya S, Lavie P. Sleep onset insomnia in sleep apnea patients: influence on acceptance of nCPAP treatment. Sleep Med 2006;7(Suppl):S85.

67. Barthlen GM, Lange DJ. Unexpectedly severe sleep and respiratory pathology in patients with amyotrophic lateral sclerosis. Eur J Neurol 2000; 7(3):299–302.

68. Weaver TE, Kribbs NB, Pack AI, et al. Night-to-night variability in CPAP use over the first three months of treatment. Sleep 1997;20(4).

69. Smith SS, Dunn N, Douglas J, et al. Sleep onset insomnia is associated with reduced adherence to CPAP therapy. Sleep Biol Rhythms 2009;7:A74.

70. Nguyên X, Chaskalovic J, Rakotonanahary D, et al. Insomnia symptoms and CPAP compliance in OSAS patients: a descriptive study using data mining methods. Sleep Med 2010;11(8):777–84.

71. Wickwire EM, Smith MT, Birnbaum S, et al. Sleep maintenance insomnia complaints predict poor CPAP adherence: a clinical case series. Sleep Med 2010;11(8):772–6.

72. Pieh C, Bach M, Popp R, et al. Insomnia symptoms influence CPAP compliance. Sleep Breath 2012; 17(1):99–104.

73. Salepci B, Caglayan B, Kiral N, et al. CPAP adherence of patients with obstructive sleep apnea. Respir Care 2013;58(9):1467–73.

74. Wallace DM, Vargas SS, Schwartz SJ, et al. Determinants of continuous positive airway pressure adherence in a sleep clinic cohort of South Florida Hispanic veterans. Sleep Breath 2013;17(1): 351–63.

75. Stepnowsky C, Zamora T, Edwards C. Does positive airway pressure therapy result in improved sleep quality? Health Psychol 2014;6:2416–24.

76. Mysliwiec V, Capaldi V, Gill J, et al. Adherence to positive airway pressure therapy in U.S. military personnel with sleep apnea improves sleepiness, sleep quality, and depressive symptoms. Mil Med 2015;180(4):475–82.

77. Wohlgemuth WK, Chirinos DA, Domingo S, et al. Attempters, adherers, and non-adherers: Latent profile analysis of CPAP use with correlates. Sleep Med 2015;16:336–42.

78. Eysteinsdottir B, Gislason T, Pack AI, et al. Insomnia complaints in lean patients with obstructive sleep apnea negatively affect positive airway pressure treatment adherence. J Sleep Res 2016; 26(2):159–65.

79. Gagnadoux F, Vaillant ML, Paris A, et al. Relationship between OSA clinical phenotypes and CPAP treatment outcomes. Chest 2016;149(1):288–90.

80. Libman E, Bailes S, Fichten CS, et al. CPAP treatment adherence in women with obstructive sleep apnea. Sleep Disord Hindawi. 2017;2017:1–8.

81. Cho YW, Kim KT, Moon H-j, et al. Comorbid insomnia with obstructive sleep apnea: clinical Characteristics and risk factors. J Clin Sleep Med 2018;14(3):409–17.

82. El-Solh AA, Adamo D, Kufel T. Comorbid insomnia and sleep apnea in Veterans with post-traumatic stress disorder. Sleep and Breathing 2018;1–9.

83. Philip P, Bioulac S, Altena E, et al. Specific insomnia symptoms and self-efficacy explain CPAP compliance in a sample of OSAS patients. PloS one 2018;13(4):e0195343.

84. Fichten C, Tran D, Rizzo D, et al. 0365 insomnia subtypes before and after Cpap treatment of sleep apnea. Sleep 2018;41(suppl_1):A140.

85. Park YK, Joo EYJJOSM. Sleep onset insomnia and depression Discourage patients from using positive airway pressure 2018;15(2):55–61.

86. Sawunyavisuth B. What are predictors for a continuous positive airway pressure machine purchasing in obstructive sleep apnea patients? Asia Pacific J Sci Technol 2018;23(3):1–5.

87. Wallace DM, Sawyer A, Shafazand S. Comorbid insomnia symptoms predict lower 6-month adherence to CPAP in US veterans with obstructive sleep apnea. Sleep and Breathing 2018;22(1):5–15.

88. Drakou T, Steiropoulos P, Saroglou M, et al. The presence of insomnia and depression contributes to the acceptance of an initial treatment trial of continuous positive airway pressure therapy in patients with obstructive sleep apnea. Sleep and Breathing 2021;25(4):1803–12.

89. Guilleminault C, Davis K, Huynh NT. Prospective randomized study of patients with insomnia and mild sleep disordered breathing. Sleep 2008;31(11):1527–33.

90. Krakow B, Melendrez D, Sisley B, et al. Nasal dilator strip therapy for chronic sleep-maintenance insomnia and symptoms of sleep-disordered breathing: a randomized controlled trial. Sleep Breath 2006;10(1):16–28.

91. Proothi M, Grazina VJ, Gold AR. Chronic insomnia remitting after maxillomandibular advancement for mild obstructive sleep apnea: a case series. J Med case Rep 2019;13(1):1–11.

92. Wallace DM, Wohlgemuth WK. 0558 Upper airway stimulation in US veterans with obstructive sleep apnea with and without insomnia: a preliminary study. Sleep 2019;42(Supplement_1):A222–3.

93. Machado MAC, De Carvalho LBC, Juliano ML, et al. Clinical comorbidities in obstructive sleep apnea syndrome treated with mandibular repositioning appliance. Respir Med 2006;100(6):988–95.

94. Carter SG, Eckert DJ. Effects of hypnotics on obstructive sleep apnea endotypes and severity: novel insights into pathophysiology and treatment. Sleep Med Rev 2021;58:101492.

95. Miller CB, Valenti L, Harrison CM, et al. Time trends in the family physician management of insomnia: the Australian experience (2000–2015). J Clin Sleep Med 2017;13(06):785–90.

96. Begum M, Gonzalez-Chica D, Bernardo C, et al. Trends in the prescription of drugs used for insomnia in Australian general practice, 2011-2018. Br J Gen Pract 2021;71(712):e877–86.

97. Sweetman A, Putland S, Lack L, et al. The effect of cognitive behavioural therapy for insomnia on sedative-hypnotic use: a narrative review. Sleep Med Rev 2020;56.

98. Royal Australian College. of General Practitioners (RACGP) Guideline document. Prescribing drugs of dependence in general practice. Part B: Benzodiazepines 2015.

99. Wilson S, Anderson K, Baldwin D, et al. British Association for Psychopharmacology consensus statement on evidence-based treatment of insomnia, parasomnias and circadian rhythm disorders: an update. J Psychopharmacol 2019;33(8):923–47.

100. Eckert DJ, White DP, Jordan AS, et al. Defining phenotypic causes of obstructive sleep apnea. Identification of novel therapeutic targets. Am J Respir Crit Care Med 2013;188(8):996–1004.

101. Zhang XJ, Li QY, Wang Y, et al. The effect of non-benzodiazepine hypnotics on sleep quality and severity in patients with OSA: a meta-analysis. Sleep and Breathing 2014;18(4):781–9.

102. Messineo L, Eckert DJ, Lim R, et al. Zolpidem increases sleep efficiency and the respiratory arousal threshold without changing sleep apnoea severity and pharyngeal muscle activity. J Physiol 2020;598(20):4681–92.

103. Cheng JY, Filippov G, Moline M, et al. Respiratory safety of lemborexant in healthy adult and elderly subjects with mild obstructive sleep apnea: a randomized, double-blind, placebo-controlled, crossover study. J Sleep Res 2020;29(4):e13021.

104. Everitt H, McDermott L, Leydon G, et al. GPs' management strategies for patients with insomnia: a survey and qualitative interview study. Br J Gen Pract 2014;64(619):e112–9.

105. Everitt H, Baldwin DS, Stuart B, et al. Antidepressants for insomnia in adults. Cochrane Database Syst Rev 2018;(5):CD010753.

106. Khazaie H, Sharafkhaneh A, Khazaie S, et al. A weight-independent association between atypical antipsychotic medications and obstructive sleep apnea. Sleep and Breathing 2018;22(1):109–14.

107. Qaseem A, Kansagara D, Forciea MA, et al. Management of chronic insomnia disorder in adults: a clinical practice guideline from the American College of Physicians. Ann Intern Med 2016;165(2):125–33.

108. Schutte-Rodin S, Broch L, Buysse D, et al. Clinical guideline for the evaluation and management of chronic insomnia in adults. J Clin Sleep Med 2008;4(5):487–504.

109. Sweetman A, Lovato N, Haycock J, et al. Improved access to effective non-drug treatment options for insomnia in Australian general practice. Med Today 2020;21(11):14–21.

110. Troxel WM, Germain A, Buysse DJ. Clinical management of insomnia with brief behavioral treatment (BBTI). Behav Sleep Med 2012;10(4):266–79.

111. Buysse DJ, Germain A, Moul DE, et al. Efficacy of brief behavioral treatment for chronic insomnia in older adults. Arch Intern Med 2011;171(10):887–95.

112. Sweetman A, Zwar N, Grivell N, et al. A step-by-step model for a brief behavioural treatment for insomnia in Australian General Practice. Aust J Gen Pract 2020;50(50):287–93.

113. Edinger JD, Simmons B, Goelz K, et al. A pilot test of an online cognitive-behaioural insomnia therapy for patients with comorbid insomnia and sleep apnea. Sleep 2015;A236. Conference Abstract Supplement(0676).

114. Sweetman A, Lack L, Catcheside P, et al. Cognitive and behavioral therapy for insomnia increases the use of continuous positive airway pressure therapy in obstructive sleep apnea participants with comorbid insomnia: a randomized clinical trial. Sleep 2019;42(12):zsz178.

115. Ong JC, Crawford MR, Dawson SC, et al. A randomized controlled trial of CBT-I and PAP for obstructive sleep apnea and comorbid insomnia: main outcomes from the MATRICS study. Sleep 2020;43(9):zsaa041.

116. Alessi CA, Fung CH, Dzierzewski JM, et al. Randomized controlled trial of an integrated approach to treating insomnia and improving use of positive airway pressure therapy in veterans with comorbid

insomnia disorder and obstructive sleep apnea. Sleep 2021;44(4):1–13.

117. Bjorvatn B, Berge T, Lehmann S, et al. No effect of a self-help book for insomnia in patients with obstructive sleep apnea and comorbid chronic insomnia–a randomized controlled trial. Front Psychol 2018;9:2413.

118. Sweetman A, McEvoy R, Smith S, et al. The effect of cognitive and behavioral therapy for insomnia on week-to-week changes in sleepiness and sleep parameters in insomnia patients with comorbid moderate and severe sleep apnea: a randomized controlled trial. Sleep 2020;43(7):zsaa002.

119. Arnedt JT, Conroy DA, Mooney A, et al. Telemedicine versus face-to-face Delivery of cognitive behavioral therapy for insomnia: a randomized controlled non-inferiority trial. Sleep 2020;44(1): zsaa136.

120. Espie CA, Kyle SD, Williams C, et al. A randomized, placebo-controlled trial of online cognitive behavioral therapy for chronic insomnia disorder delivered via an automated media-rich web application. Sleep 2012;35(6):769–81.

121. Soh HL, Ho RC, Ho CS, et al. Efficacy of digital cognitive behavioural therapy for insomnia: a meta-analysis of randomised controlled trials. Sleep Med 2020;75:315–25.

122. Ye Y-y, Zhang Y-f, Chen J, et al. Internet-based cognitive behavioral therapy for insomnia (ICBT-i) improves comorbid anxiety and depression—a meta-analysis of randomized controlled trials. PLoS One 2015;10(11):e0142258.

123. Mercer JD, Bootzin RR, Lack L. Insomniacs' perception of wake instead of sleep. Sleep 2002; 25(5):559–66.

124. Bonnet MH, Arand DL. Hyperarousal and insomnia: state of the science. Sleep Med Rev 2010;14(1): 9–15.

125. Ratnavadivel R, Chau N, Stadler D, et al. Marked reduction in obstructive sleep apnea severity in slow wave sleep. J Clin Sleep Med 2009;5(6): 519–24.

126. Riemann D, Spiegelhalder K, Nissen C, et al. REM sleep instability–a new pathway for insomnia? Pharmacopsychiatry 2012;45(05):167–76.

127. Krakow B, Romero E, Ulibarri VA, et al. Prospective assessment of nocturnal awakenings in a case series of treatment-seeking chronic insomnia patients: a pilot study of subjective and objective causes. Sleep 2012;35(12):1685–92.

128. Sériès F, Roy N, Marc I. Effects of sleep deprivation and sleep fragmentation on upper airway collapsibility in normal subjects. Am J Respir Crit Care Med 1994;150(2):481–5.

129. Persson HE, Svanborg E. Sleep deprivation worsens obstructive sleep apnea: Comparison between diurnal and nocturnal polysomnography. Chest 1996;109(3):645–50.

130. Benetó A, Gomez-Siurana E, Rubio-Sanchez P. Comorbidity between sleep apnea and insomnia. Sleep Med Rev 2009;13(4):287–93.

131. Sweetman. Association of co-morbid insomnia and sleep apnoea symptoms with all-cause mortality: Analysis of the NHANES 2005-2008 data, Sleep Epidemiology 2022. in press.

## FURTHER READING

Sweetman A, Lechat B, Appleton A, Reynolds A, Adams R, Melaku YA. Association of co-morbid insomnia and sleep apnoea symptoms with all-cause mortality: Analysis of the NHANES 2005-2008 data. Sleep Epidemiology 2022. In press.

# Obstructive Sleep Apnea and Positive Airway Pressure Usage in Populations with Neurological Disease

Daniel A. Barone, MD*, Alan Z. Segal, MD

## KEYWORDS

- OSA • CPAP • Stroke • Cognition • Epilepsy • Migraine

## KEY POINTS

- Obstructive sleep apnea (OSA) is a very common condition that can negatively affect and/or precipitate multiple neurologic conditions including stroke, cognition, epilepsy, and migraines.
- Treatment with continuous positive airway pressure (CPAP) can improve not only overall health and quality of life in those with OSA but also may positively affect the aforementioned neurologic domains.
- Screening and/or workup for OSA should be considered in any neurologic patient who presents with stroke, cognitive decline, epilepsy, and/or migraines/headaches.

## INTRODUCTION

Obstructive sleep apnea (OSA) is characterized by repetitive episodes of complete or partial upper airway obstruction during sleep, with a worldwide estimate of 936 million sufferers.[1] Treatments of OSA include continuous positive airway pressure (CPAP), weight loss, positional therapy, oral appliances, positive upper airway pressure, oromaxillofacial surgery, hypoglossal nerve stimulation, bariatric surgery, and others,[2] with CPAP being the most commonly prescribed treatment.[3] In this review, the neurologic conditions of stroke, cognitive decline, epilepsy, and migraines will be discussed because they relate to OSA. Additionally, the literature regarding improvement in these conditions following treatment with CPAP will be explored.

## STROKE

### Relationship Between Obstructive Sleep Apnea and Stroke

The relationship between OSA and stroke can be best understood in the context of a broad spectrum of cardiovascular outcomes including hypertension, coronary artery disease, heart failure, and atrial fibrillation.[4–7] Furthermore, untreated OSA has been significantly associated with an increase in cardiovascular and cerebrovascular mortality. The mechanism by which these effects occur is not fully understood but it has been postulated that recurrent hypoxic events in OSA leads to increased inflammation, sympathetic activation, and the formation of free radicals. As a result, there may be dysfunction of the endothelium, platelet aggregation and changes in cerebral blood flow. Multiple observational studies and cross-sectional population analyses have shown an association between OSA and stroke but given the common vascular risk factors shared with cardiovascular disease in general, it can be difficult to tease out a specific effect as opposed to shared vascular risk factors.[8–10]

In 2005, a landmark study by Yaggi and colleagues demonstrated that OSA is an independent risk factor for stroke, even after thoroughly adjusting for comorbidities.[11] In this prospective cohort, all aged older than 50 years, a 2-fold risk of stroke was found in patients with OSA as compared with

Weill Cornell Center for Sleep Medicine, Weill Cornell Medicine | NewYork-Presbyterian, 425 East 61st Street, 5th floor, New York, NY 10065, USA
* Corresponding author.
E-mail address: dab9129@med.cornell.edu

Sleep Med Clin 17 (2022) 619–627
https://doi.org/10.1016/j.jsmc.2022.07.007
1556-407X/22/© 2022 Elsevier Inc. All rights reserved.

controls. Although a subset of OSA patients were treated with CPAP, there was a persistent risk of stroke, likely representing vascular injury before the initiation of CPAP or possibly due to lack of adherence to CPAP, a factor that has impeded demonstration of the benefit of this treatment in heart failure cohorts.

There is also data to show that OSA can occur as a result of stroke. Insults to the central nervous system may result in changes in breathing patterns or possibly unmask previously undiagnosed pre-stroke OSA in the poststroke period.[12] Prevalence of OSA in patients with a history of stroke has been shown to be as high as 62%.[13] The stroke–OSA association may be uniquely associated with strokes that occur in the early morning or produce a "wake-up" from sleep,[14,15] suggesting that acute changes during sleep such as hypoxia, acute elevations in blood pressure, or other hemodynamic changes are acute precipitants of a cerebrovascular event. In poststroke patients, the diagnosis of OSA is associated with worse neurologic outcomes.[16]

Diagnosis of OSA in patients who have had a stroke can be challenging due to limitations posed by neurologic deficits and the complex logistical challenges posed by poststroke rehabilitation and hospitalization. Adherence to CPAP in post-stroke patients can be suboptimal and is significantly poorer that in the general population receiving an OSA diagnosis and CPAP treatment.[15]

### Effect of Treatment with Continuous Positive Airway Pressure on Stroke

CPAP should be the primary treatment modality for the prevention of stroke in patients with OSA. Along with CPAP, attention should also be paid to lifestyle changes, such as weight loss, diet, and exercise. In a meta-analysis of 7 trials assessing the effectiveness of lifestyle interventions in OSA, it was shown that control of these modifiable risks showed a significant pooled mean reduction in apnea-hypopnea index (AHI) of 6.0/h.[17]

Multiple studies have shown evidence that CPAP therapy can effectively prevent stroke. One small study, with long-term follow-up of 168 patients treated with CPAP, showed that cardiovascular outcomes, including stroke showed a significant risk reduction from 15% to 2% during 7.5 years of follow-up.[18] In a larger observational study in men, the 10-year incidence of cardiovascular events (stroke and myocardial infarction), the event rate was 0.35 per 100 person years when on CPAP, compared with 1.06 in untreated patients, a 3-fold reduction.[4] In contrast to men, 2 prospective cohort studies in women suggested a trend toward CPAP benefit. Although not statistically significant, risk of cardiovascular events showed hazard ratios in the 2.8 to 3.5 range, an effect that was even more pronounced for stroke specifically, with a hazard ratio of 6.4.[19] With the use of CPAP, hazard ratios decreased into the 0.55 to 0.91 range but this effect did not reach statistical significance in either study. In a meta-analysis of 9 trials assessing the effects of CPAP on prevention of cardiovascular events and mortality in patients with OSA, the relative risk of stroke was reduced, with a relative risk of 0.77.[20]

Despite the evidence above, the results of the Sleep Apnea Cardiovascular Endpoints (SAVE) trial[21] led to some controversy in this arena. It included 2717 patients from 89 sites in 7 countries, and surprisingly failed to show improvement in cardiovascular endpoints such as stroke and myocardial infarction. Participants had moderate-to-severe OSA without daytime sleepiness, with 80% being men, and average CPAP adherence of 3.3 hours per night; the mean AHI on CPAP was 3.7/h, decreased from 29.0/h at baseline. After an average follow-up of 3.7 years, there was no effect on any individual or other composite cardiovascular outcome. However, there was a trend toward a lower risk of stroke for those with good CPAP adherence (hazard ratio, 0.56; 95% CI, 0.32–1.00; $P = .05$), as well as a lower risk of the composite endpoint of cerebral events (hazard ratio, 0.52; 95% CI, 0.30–0.90; $P = .02$). As indicated above, previous data suggested that OSA in adults carried a markedly increased risk of adverse cardiovascular events, and that CPAP treatment might ameliorate that risk. Considerable discussion has occurred since the publication of the SAVE primary findings as to the possible reasons for the neutral cardiovascular result[22] including the fact that, on average, patients used CPAP for only about half the night (ie, 3.3 hours), raising the possibility that had they been able to use the treatment longer, a treatment benefit may have been observed.[23]

Regardless, the effect of CPAP therapy in patients with OSA, although effective in stroke prevention generally, may be even more effective with regard to specific stroke mechanisms. Atrial fibrillation, an important cause of stroke, that can often be occult, is more prevalent in patients with OSA, and the treatment of OSA may allow maintenance of sinus rhythm in patients undergoing cardioversion. In paroxysmal atrial fibrillation, it has been shown that the duration of time spent in sinus rhythm compared with AF can be directly correlated with fluctuations in sleep-disordered breathing (SDB).[24] Another stroke risk factor, carotid artery atherosclerotic disease, is more common in both snorers and patients with OSA. In addition to the known risks of atherosclerosis associated with OSA, it has been postulated that the vibrational effects of snoring and OSA may promote increased vascular turbulence and promote plaque progression in cervical vessels.[25]

In poststroke recovery and secondary prevention, there is mixed data that the use of CPAP may improve outcomes. In one study of 166 patients, only 28 tolerated and were still using CPAP at 5-year follow-up. Lack of CPAP therapy in this cohort was further associated with poststroke mortality and stroke severity.[26] Functionally, early institution of CPAP therapy (3–6 days after stroke onset) has been shown to accelerate neurologic recovery and improve functional outcomes, as measured by the modified Rankin disability score.[27] A meta-analysis of 10 randomized controlled trials examining CPAP in poststroke patients showed an overall increase in functional and cognitive improvement but there was a significant attrition of CPAP use over time. These data suggest that the treatment of OSA with CPAP in the poststroke setting is important to achieve short-term stroke recovery, even if long-term secondary stroke prevention may not be achieved. It has also been shown that CPAP adherence was greater in patients with greater poststroke functional capacity in comparison to those more severely disabled suggesting that the CPAP treatment of OSA in poststroke patients may not be used in the patients who could derive the greatest therapeutic benefit.[28]

## COGNITION
### Effect of Obstructive Sleep Apnea on Cognition

The association between OSA and neurocognitive impairment has been evaluated through multiple data sets[3]; potential factors accounting for this association include chronic intermittent hypoxia as the most likely explanation,[29] as well as the presence of anxiety or depression, lack of quality sleep/sleep fragmentation, and excessive daytime sleepiness.[30] Additionally, it has been shown that depressive and anxious symptoms are found in those with OSA at 35%.[31] A recent meta-analysis demonstrated that the presence of Alzheimer disease (AD) presents a 5-fold increased risk of OSA, and that roughly 50% of AD patients experience OSA.[32] Finally, OSA seems to be an independent risk factor for cognitive decline in older patients,[33] and OSA is prevalent in 27% of patients with mild cognitive impairment (MCI).[34]

OSA may result in significant detriment across several neurologic and cognitive domains, with the greatest impact on attention, vigilance, and information processing speed, as well as on the development and progression of MCI. Treatment with CPAP seems to mitigate and slow the rate of cognitive decline and may reduce the risk of dementia but larger prospective studies will be required to further elucidate the full scope of this effect.[3]

In a review of 17 studies investigating structural brain alteration and cognitive impairment in OSA, it was noted that those with OSA had worse performance in attention, memory, and executive function compared with healthy controls; additionally, it was demonstrated that cognitive impairment was associated with OSA severity, with treatment able to improve certain cognitive domains.[35] Similarly, in a meta-analysis of 19,940 participants from 6 cohort studies examining the association between SDB and cognition demonstrated that adults with SDB were at significantly higher risk of cognitive decline, with women having greater risk than men.[33]

In one study testing cognitive function in 1084 adults with suspected OSA, several parameters of cognition were analyzed including the Montreal Cognitive Assessment Test. About 48% of all patients met the threshold for MCI, which increased to greater than 55% in those with moderate-to-severe OSA; those with moderate and severe OSA were associated with greater than 70% higher odds of having MCI. Additionally, those with OSA presented reduced episodic memory and information processing speed, with processing speed decreasing with increasing OSA severity.[36]

A meta-analysis was performed on the effects of OSA and role of CPAP on executive function, and it was found that all components of executive function were impaired by the presence of OSA, and that executive function did improve modestly with the treatment with CPAP, whereas age and OSA severity did not modulate the effects of these changes.[37]

A study with 32 patients with moderate-to-severe OSA was performed using a computerized battery demonstrated that these patients suffer deficits in various attention processes.[38] In another study, impaired vigilance as well as decreased tonic alertness and an impairment of simulated driving performance was noted in those with OSA as compared with controls.[39] Similarly, another study demonstrated that obesity is a risk factor for impaired vigilance in those with OSA. Patients with OSA and obesity compared with non-obese OSA patients were noted to have delayed reaction times and a decrease in working memory.[40] Finally, a third study showed that factors associated with vigilance-related cognitive decline were shown to include OSA severity, change in oxygen desaturation, and sleep fragmentation.[41]

Cognitive impairment has been associated with EEG slowing, and in those with OSA and obesity hypoventilation syndrome (OHS), a study was performed showing that those with OHS demonstrate greater slow frequency electroencephalogram activity, as compared with equally obese OSA patients. Moreover, those with OHS have greater slow frequency EEG activity during sleep and wake than equally obese patients with OSA, and greater EEG slowing was associated with worse vigilance and lower oxygenation during sleep.[42]

### Effect of Treatment with Continuous Positive Airway Pressure on Cognition

The Apnea Positive Pressure Long-term Efficacy Study was a 6-month, randomized, double-blind, 2-arm, sham-controlled, and multicenter trial and demonstrated that CPAP usage resulted in mild, transient improvement in the most sensitive measures of executive and frontal-lobe function for those with severe OSA.[43]

A meta-analysis of randomized controlled trials on the cognitive effects of CPAP for OSA was performed, with 14 trials and 1926 patients, and discovered that CPAP usage can partially improve cognitive impairment in the population of severe OSA, especially in attention and information processing speed.[44]

Short-term effects of CPAP demonstrated mixed findings as per recent studies. In a study of 182 patients with mild-to-severe OSA, no predictive relationship between subjective improvements in daytime sleepiness, fatigue, and depression, and objective vigilance with CPAP usage was found in patients with OSA.[45] In another, a sample of 16 patients with moderate-to-severe OSA, who were assessed both before and after 3 months of CPAP treatment, there were significant improvements in executive functions and memory but no significant changes in mood, anxiety, aggressive behavior, and quality of life.[46] In another study, a cross-sectional, prospective observational study of 126 patients, 3 months of CPAP treatment alleviated daytime sleepiness, as well as depressive and anxiety symptoms but there was no significant improvement in cognitive performance.[47]

Using a large retrospective analysis, associations between CPAP therapy, adherence, and incident diagnoses of AD, MCI, and dementia not-otherwise-specified in older adults were evaluated. Using Medicare claims data of 53,321 beneficiaries with an OSA diagnosis, it was found that CPAP treatment and adherence were independently associated with lower odds of incident AD diagnoses in older adults, suggesting that the treatment of OSA may reduce the risk of subsequent dementia.[48]

Two recent studies evaluated the long-term effects of CPAP use and MCI. In one, CPAP adherence on cognition in older adults with mild OSA and MCI was evaluated; there were 2 groups—the CPAP adherent group with MCI with an average CPAP use of 4 hours or greater per night and a CPAP nonadherent group with MCI with an average CPAP use of less than 4 hours per night. Those who were adherent demonstrated a significant improvement in psychomotor/cognitive processing speed.[49] In another study, 1-year use of CPAP in adults with OSA and MCI was evaluated. It was demonstrated that CPAP adherence in patients with MCI significantly improved cognition and possibly slowed cognitive decline.[50]

The benefit of CPAP on cognitive performance is not universal throughout the medical literature. In a retrospective review comparing 96 patients during a period of 2.8 years with MCI and OSA that were either CPAP compliant, CPAP noncompliant, or not on CPAP treatment, the use of CPAP was not associated with delay in progression to dementia or cognitive decline.[51] In a systemic review and meta-analysis on the effects of CPAP compared with mandibular advancement device (MAD), no significant differences between MAD and CPAP in quality of life, cognitive, and functional outcomes were found but the results may have been limited by low treatment compliance.[52]

There seems to be evidence that CPAP therapy may improve cognitive function or slow the progression to MCI and AD in those with OSA but large longitudinal studies demonstrating this are lacking. Studies that evaluate cognitive function and the use of CPAP are limited, and most do not attempt to explain the cause of the cognitive findings by imaging, biomarkers, or PSG data.[3]

## EPILEPSY
### Relationship Between Obstructive Sleep Apnea and Epilepsy

It is well-known that the presence of OSA exhibits a high comorbidity with epilepsy.[53] In patients with OSA, the termination of apneic spells is associated with transient arousals,[54] leading to marked disruption and fragmentation of normal sleep, ultimately resulting in sleep deprivation.[53] In animal models, sleep deprivation has been shown to increase the susceptibility to seizures.[55,56] In patients with epilepsy, several studies have reported increased seizure frequency following sleep deprivation.[57,58] Others have directly implicated sleep deprivation and sleep fragmentation in the increased incidence of epilepsy in patients with OSA.[59–61]

Severity of epilepsy has a relationship with OSA; in those with epilepsy and OSA, the frequency of seizures is increased compared with those with epilepsy without OSA.[62] Those with refractory epilepsy consist of approximately 30% of all epileptic patients,[63] and in these patients, the prevalence of OSA has been estimated to be 33%.[64] In one study, a higher prevalence of OSA (43.8%) was reported in those (n = 32) with severe refractory epilepsy (>1 seizure per month) as compared with 30.7% of the 52 in the mild group (0–1 seizures per month).[65] In a different study, a higher prevalence (4 out of 20) of OSA was found in those with refractory epilepsy as compared with none in the controlled epilepsy group.[66]

In one study featuring 480 adults with OSA, 4% were reported to have seizures[67]; in another study including 139 young children with OSA (age range 0–17 months), 17% were reported to have epilepsy as a comorbidity.[68] Demonstrating the bidirectionality of this relationship, a meta-analysis of 26 studies of patients with epilepsy showed that roughly 33% had OSA, with OSA being present in those with focal seizures at 32.2%, and in those with generalized seizures at 28.2%.[69]

In those with OSA, apneic events due to upper airway obstruction can occur in both rapid eye movement (REM) and non-REM (NREM) sleep, but are more frequent,[70] and are of longer duration during REM sleep as compared with NREM sleep.[71] Sleep architecture becomes fragmented in OSA due to repeated arousals and microarousals, and results in poor sleep quality.[72] These arousals in REM can potentially restart the sleep cycle, which may result in shorter REM periods and decreased total REM time[53]; similarly, increases in NREM stage 1 (N1) and N2 sleep with a corresponding decrease in REM has been reported in those with OSA.[73] This is significant due to the fact that cortical activity is synchronized during NREM sleep but desynchronized during REM sleep and wakefulness,[74] which serves to reduce electrographic seizures during REM sleep and wakefulness.[75] As such, a review of 42 studies with 1458 patients demonstrated that REM sleep has been reported as the most protective stage of sleep against seizures.[74]

Although quality sleep is definitely important for epilepsy patients, those with OSA demonstrate increased sleep-stage transitions, which may alter the time spent in certain sleep stages without affecting the overall amounts of each sleep stage or total sleep time. This, in combination with reduced REM sleep and increased REM sleep fragmentation as above, negatively affects seizure threshold in OSA patients.[76,77]

## Effect of Treatment with Continuous Positive Airway Pressure on Epilepsy

Multiple studies have demonstrated an improvement in seizure control after treatment in those with both OSA and epilepsy.[59,78,79] REM sleep is affected predominantly in those with OSA, resulting in decreased REM time and increased fragmentation of REM sleep, thus resulting in poor quality.[80] Following this REM sleep deprivation, a phenomenon known as REM rebound can be seen in patients with OSA on treatment; one meta-analysis, which included 14 studies with 119 patients of OSA, REM rebound occurred with REM sleep time increasing from 13.8% to 20.0%, corresponding to a 57% relative increase in REM sleep time, during CPAP titration as compared with baseline PSG.[53] CPAP also resulted in improved architecture in terms of decreased sleep fragmentation.[53,81]

Studies of patients with OSA following treatment with CPAP have shown occurrence of transient rebound REM sleep and an increase in REM density,[82,83] as well as better seizure control — a significant number of cases have been reported to even become seizure free.[78] In patients with OSA and drug-resistant epilepsy, treatment with CPAP has also been shown to improve sleep architecture (increased REM sleep/density), and although there does not exist any randomized control trials, anecdotal reports suggest that CPAP treatment alone may improve seizure control in this group of patients; authors have noted that such a noninvasive treatment can be an effective adjunctive therapy, potentially eliminating the requirement of invasive and expensive interventions.[53]

Disruption and/or deprivation of REM sleep seems to be an important factor in the development of drug-resistant epilepsy given its importance in the development of improved seizure control in patients with OSA and epilepsy when being treated with CPAP.[53] Thus, restoring normal sleep architecture is paramount in patients with epilepsy, and screening for disturbances in sleep architecture (and judicious use of sleep testing) therefore should be an essential component of epilepsy management.[53]

## MIGRAINE
### Relationship Between Obstructive Sleep Apnea and Migraine

Headache on awakening from sleep is a known historical clue to the presence of OSA in patients undergoing sleep evaluation. Although the precise mechanism is not known, it has been hypothesized that a decrease in oxygenation, along with vasodilation from increased carbon dioxide may serve to precipitate pain.[84] Alternatively, OSA-associated sleep fragmentation may create a decrease in pain thresholds and an increase in spontaneous pain.[85] Even in the absence of documented OSA, snoring on a population basis has been consistently associated with headache disorders.[86] Obesity is a known risk factor for both headache and SDB.[87]

OSA is associated with multiple types of headaches including, headaches on awakening, tension headache, cluster headache, and migraine.[88] Although migraine among headache disorders is best understood to be a cerebrovascular disorder, on a population basis, the prevalence of OSA is similar when comparing patients with migraine as compared with the general population.[89] Moreover, OSA is equally prevalent comparing patients with migraine without and with aura, a phenomenon at least partially attributable to vasoconstriction followed by vasodilation.[90] Mechanistically, the relationship between migraine and sleep may relate to serotonin because it is known that increases in this transmitter may explain migraine and is known to be a disruptor of REM sleep. Wake-up or alarm clock headaches, are thought to be a REM phenomenon and are more common in patients with OSA.[88] Conversely to serotonin, dopamine levels may be decreased both in patients with migraine and with OSA.[91]

Mood disorders may also serve to link headache syndromes with OSA. Headache is increased in patients with depression, and there may be a relationship between depression and OSA, suggesting a common pathophysiology.[92] Anxiety is known to increase the incidence of tension headaches, and OSA-associated sleep disruption has been shown to promote muscle spasm and associated tension headache.[93]

### Effect of Treatment with Continuous Positive Airway Pressure on Migraine

The role of sleep in aborting a migraine headache, as well as headache in general, is commonly recognized but not specifically explained. In animal models, it has been hypothesized that this benefit may be related to the so-called glymphatic system, which clears the brain of toxins during sleep. In mice, Schain and colleagues, demonstrated that cortical spreading depression (known to occur in migraine) precipitates the closing of gap junctions and impairment of glymphatic function.[94]

With specific regard to OSA and migraine, treatment with CPAP has a favorable effect on migraine, as studies have shown an improvement in sleep quality, associated with a reduction in migraine frequency (from 5.8 to 0.4 attacks per month). Moreover, duration of migraine decreased from an average of 22 hours to 3 hours. There was a decrease in lost workdays (from 1.2 to 0.3 per month), and there was a reduction in acute medication intake.[95] In PSG studies, improvements in migraine with the use of CPAP have been correlated with significant decreases in AHI, as well as promoting sleep quality indicators such as quantity of slow wave sleep and sleep efficiency.[96]

## SUMMARY

OSA can negatively affect multiple neurologic parameters including cognition, and can precipitate or worsen stroke, epilepsy, and migraines; as such, screening and/or workup for OSA should be considered in any neurologic patient who presents with stroke, cognitive decline, epilepsy, and/or migraines/headaches. Fortunately, treatment with CPAP can improve not only overall health and quality of life in those with OSA but it also may positively affect the aforementioned neurologic domains.

## CLINICS CARE POINTS

- When a neurologic patient presents with stroke, cognitive decline, epilepsy, and/or migraines/headaches, consideration for the possibility of OSA is an important aspect of care.
- Treatment with CPAP and/or other modalities should be started on neurologic patients with OSA as soon as possible, and regular monitoring of compliance and effectiveness is paramount.

## DISCLOSURE

Nothing of relevance to this topic.

## REFERENCES

1. Benjafield AV, et al. Estimation of the global prevalence and burden of obstructive sleep apnoea: a literature-based analysis. Lancet Respir Med 2019; 7(8):687–98.
2. Gottlieb DJ, Punjabi NM. Diagnosis and management of obstructive sleep apnea: a review. Jama 2020;323(14):1389–400.

3. Seda G, Matwiyoff G, Parrish JS. Effects of obstructive sleep apnea and CPAP on cognitive function. Curr Neurol Neurosci Rep 2021;21(7):32.

4. Marin JM, et al. Long-term cardiovascular outcomes in men with obstructive sleep apnoea-hypopnoea with or without treatment with continuous positive airway pressure: an observational study. Lancet 2005;365(9464):1046–53.

5. Gami AS, et al. Association of atrial fibrillation and obstructive sleep apnea. Circulation 2004;110(4):364–7.

6. Shahar E, et al. Sleep-disordered breathing and cardiovascular disease: cross-sectional results of the Sleep Heart Health Study. Am J Respir Crit Care Med 2001;163(1):19–25.

7. Arzt M, et al. Association of sleep-disordered breathing and the occurrence of stroke. Am J Respir Crit Care Med 2005;172(11):1447–51.

8. Bradley TD, Floras JS. Sleep apnea and heart failure: Part I: obstructive sleep apnea. Circulation 2003;107(12):1671–8.

9. Marshall NS, et al. Sleep apnea and 20-year follow-up for all-cause mortality, stroke, and cancer incidence and mortality in the Busselton Health Study cohort. J Clin Sleep Med 2014;10(4):355–62.

10. Budhiraja R, Parthasarathy S, Quan SF. Endothelial dysfunction in obstructive sleep apnea. J Clin Sleep Med 2007;3(4):409–15.

11. Yaggi HK, et al. Obstructive sleep apnea as a risk factor for stroke and death. N Engl J Med 2005;353(19):2034–41.

12. Hermann DM, Bassetti CL. Role of sleep-disordered breathing and sleep-wake disturbances for stroke and stroke recovery. Neurology 2016;87(13):1407–16.

13. Dong R, et al. Prevalence, risk factors, outcomes, and treatment of obstructive sleep apnea in patients with cerebrovascular disease: a systematic review. J Stroke Cerebrovasc Dis 2018;27(6):1471–80.

14. Hsieh SW, et al. Obstructive sleep apnea linked to wake-up strokes. J Neurol 2012;259(7):1433–9.

15. Johnson KG, Johnson DC. Frequency of sleep apnea in stroke and TIA patients: a meta-analysis. J Clin Sleep Med 2010;6(2):131–7.

16. Koo BB, et al. Observational study of obstructive sleep apnea in wake-up stroke: the SLEEP TIGHT study. Cerebrovasc Dis 2016;41(5–6):233–41.

17. Molnar MZ, et al. Association of incident obstructive sleep apnoea with outcomes in a large cohort of US veterans. Thorax 2015;70(9):888–95.

18. Doherty LS, et al. Long-term effects of nasal continuous positive airway pressure therapy on cardiovascular outcomes in sleep apnea syndrome. Chest 2005;127(6):2076–84.

19. Campos-Rodriguez F, et al. Cardiovascular mortality in women with obstructive sleep apnea with or without continuous positive airway pressure treatment: a cohort study. Ann Intern Med 2012;156(2):115–22.

20. Aaronson JA, et al. Effects of continuous positive airway pressure on cognitive and functional outcome of stroke patients with obstructive sleep apnea: a randomized controlled trial. J Clin Sleep Med 2016;12(4):533–41.

21. McEvoy RD, et al. CPAP for prevention of cardiovascular events in obstructive sleep apnea. N Engl J Med 2016;375(10):919–31.

22. Mokhlesi B, Ayas NT. Cardiovascular events in obstructive sleep apnea - can CPAP therapy SAVE Lives? N Engl J Med 2016;375(10):994–6.

23. Qiu ZH, Luo YM, McEvoy RD. The Sleep Apnea Cardiovascular Endpoints (SAVE) study: implications for health services and sleep research in China and elsewhere. J Thorac Dis 2017;9(8):2217–20.

24. Marulanda-Londono E, Chaturvedi S. The Interplay between obstructive sleep apnea and atrial fibrillation. Front Neurol 2017;8:668.

25. Lee SA, et al. Heavy snoring as a cause of carotid artery atherosclerosis. Sleep 2008;31(9):1207–13.

26. Brill AK, et al. CPAP as treatment of sleep apnea after stroke: a meta-analysis of randomized trials. Neurology 2018;90(14):e1222–30.

27. Epstein LJ, et al. Clinical guideline for the evaluation, management and long-term care of obstructive sleep apnea in adults. J Clin Sleep Med 2009;5(3):263–76.

28. Weaver EM, Maynard C, Yueh B. Survival of veterans with sleep apnea: continuous positive airway pressure versus surgery. Otolaryngol Head Neck Surg 2004;130(6):659–65.

29. Prabhakar NR, Peng Y-J, Nanduri J. Hypoxia-inducible factors and obstructive sleep apnea. J Clin Invest 2020;130(10):5042–51.

30. Liu S, et al. EEG Power spectral analysis of Abnormal cortical activations during REM/NREM sleep in obstructive sleep apnea. Front Neurol 2021;12:643855.

31. Garbarino S, et al. Association of anxiety and depression in obstructive sleep apnea patients: a systematic review and meta-analysis. Behav Sleep Med 2020;18(1):35–57.

32. Emamian F, et al. The association between obstructive sleep apnea and Alzheimer's disease: a meta-analysis Perspective. Front Aging Neurosci 2016;8:78.

33. Zhu X, Zhao Y. Sleep-disordered breathing and the risk of cognitive decline: a meta-analysis of 19,940 participants. Sleep and Breathing 2018;22(1):165–73.

34. Mubashir T, et al. The prevalence of obstructive sleep apnea in mild cognitive impairment: a systematic review. BMC Neurol 2019;19(1):195.

35. Caporale M, et al. Cognitive impairment in obstructive sleep apnea syndrome: a descriptive review. Sleep Breath 2021;25(1):29–40.

36. Beaudin AE, et al. Cognitive function in a sleep Clinic cohort of patients with obstructive sleep apnea. Ann Am Thorac Soc 2021;18(5):865–75.

37. Olaithe M, Bucks RS. Executive dysfunction in OSA before and after treatment: a meta-analysis. Sleep 2013;36(9):1297–305.

38. Angelelli P, et al. The neuropsychological Profile of attention deficits of patients with obstructive sleep apnea: an update on the daytime attentional impairment. Brain Sci 2020;10(6):325.

39. Huang Y, et al. The psychomotor vigilance test compared to a divided attention steering simulation in patients with moderate or severe obstructive sleep apnea. Nat Sci Sleep 2020;12:509–24.

40. Shen Y-C, et al. The impact of obesity in cognitive and memory dysfunction in obstructive sleep apnea syndrome. Int J Obes 2019;43(2):355–61.

41. McCloy K, et al. Polysomnographic risk factors for vigilance-related cognitive decline and obstructive sleep apnea. Sleep Breath 2021;25(1):75–83.

42. Sivam S, et al. Slow-frequency electroencephalography activity during wake and sleep in obesity hypoventilation syndrome. Sleep 2019;43(2).

43. Kushida CA, et al. Effects of continuous positive airway pressure on neurocognitive function in obstructive sleep apnea patients: the apnea positive pressure long-term Efficacy study (APPLES). Sleep 2012;35(12):1593–602.

44. Wang ML, et al. Cognitive effects of treating obstructive sleep apnea: a meta-analysis of randomized controlled trials. J Alzheimers Dis 2020;75(3):705–15.

45. Bhat S, et al. The relationships between improvements in daytime sleepiness, fatigue and depression and psychomotor vigilance task testing with CPAP use in patients with obstructive sleep apnea. Sleep Med 2018;49:81–9.

46. Turner K, et al. Obstructive sleep apnea: neurocognitive and behavioral functions before and after treatment. Funct Neurol 2019;34(2):71–8.

47. Dostálová V, et al. Effects of continuous positive airway pressure on neurocognitive and neuropsychiatric function in obstructive sleep apnea. J Sleep Res 2019;28(5):e12761.

48. Dunietz GL, et al. Obstructive sleep apnea treatment and dementia risk in older adults. Sleep 2021;44(9): zsab076.

49. Wang Y, et al. One Year of continuous positive airway pressure adherence improves cognition in older adults with mild apnea and mild cognitive impairment. Nurs Res 2020;69(2):157–64.

50. Richards KC, et al. CPAP adherence may slow 1-year cognitive decline in older adults with mild cognitive impairment and apnea. J Am Geriatr Soc 2019;67(3):558–64.

51. Skiba V, et al. Use of positive airway pressure in mild cognitive impairment to delay progression to dementia. J Clin Sleep Med 2020;16(6):863–70.

52. Schwartz M, et al. Effects of CPAP and mandibular advancement device treatment in obstructive sleep apnea patients: a systematic review and meta-analysis. Sleep and Breathing 2018;22(3):555–68.

53. Jaseja H, Goyal M, Mishra P. Drug-resistant epilepsy and obstructive sleep apnea: Exploring a link between the two. World Neurosurg 2021;146: 210–4.

54. Park JG, Ramar K, Olson EJ. Updates on definition, Consequences, and management of obstructive sleep apnea. Mayo Clinic Proc 2011;86(6):549–55.

55. Shouse MN, Sterman MB. Acute sleep deprivation reduces amygdala-kindled seizure thresholds in cats. Exp Neurol 1982;78(3):716–27.

56. Shouse MN. Sleep deprivation increases susceptibility to kindled and penicillin seizure events during all waking and sleep states in cats. Sleep 1988; 11(2):162–71.

57. Bennett DR. Sleep deprivation and major motor convulsions. Neurology 1963;13(11):953–8.

58. Gunderson CH, Dunne PB, Feyer TL. Sleep deprivation seizures. Neurology 1973;23(7):678–86.

59. Vaughn BV, et al. Improvement of epileptic seizure control with treatment of obstructive sleep apnoea. Seizure 1996;5(1):73–8.

60. Nishimura Y, et al. Ictal central apnea and bradycardia in temporal lobe epilepsy complicated by obstructive sleep apnea syndrome. Epilepsy Behav Case Rep 2015;4:41–4.

61. Ferini-Strambi L, et al. Neurological deficits in obstructive sleep apnea. Curr Treat Options Neurol 2017;19(4):16.

62. Shaheen HA, et al. Obstructive sleep apnea in epilepsy: a preliminary Egyptian study. Sleep and Breathing 2012;16(3):765–71.

63. Kalilani L, et al. The epidemiology of drug-resistant epilepsy: a systematic review and meta-analysis. Epilepsia 2018;59(12):2179–93.

64. Malow BA, et al. Obstructive sleep apnea is common in medically refractory epilepsy patients. Neurology 2000;55(7):1002–7.

65. Jain SV, et al. Obstructive sleep apnea in children with epilepsy: prospective pilot trial. Acta Neurol Scand 2012;125(1):e3–6.

66. Zanzmera P, et al. Markedly disturbed sleep in medically refractory compared to controlled epilepsy - a clinical and polysomnography study. Seizure 2012; 21(7):487–90.

67. Sonka K, et al. Seizures in sleep apnea patients: occurrence and time distribution. Sb Lek 2000; 101(3):229–32.

68. Qubty WF, et al. Comorbidities in Infants with obstructive sleep apnea. J Clin Sleep Med 2014; 10(11):1213–6.

69. Lin Z, Si Q, Xiaoyi Z. Obstructive sleep apnoea in patients with epilepsy: a meta-analysis. Sleep and Breathing 2017;21(2):263–70.

70. Ho ML, Brass SD. Obstructive sleep apnea. Neurol Int 2011;3(3):e15.

71. Goh DY, Galster P, Marcus CL. Sleep architecture and respiratory disturbances in children with obstructive sleep apnea. Am J Respir Crit Care Med 2000;162(2 Pt 1):682–6.

72. Sullivan CE, Issa FG. Pathophysiological mechanisms in obstructive sleep apnea. Sleep 1980;3(3–4):235–46.

73. Basunia M, et al. Relationship of symptoms with sleep-stage abnormalities in obstructive sleep apnea-hypopnea syndrome. J Community Hosp Intern Med Perspect 2016;6(4):32170.

74. Ng M, Pavlova M. Why are seizures rare in rapid eye movement sleep? Review of the frequency of seizures in different sleep stages. Epilepsy Res Treat 2013;2013:932790.

75. Shouse MN, Farber PR, Staba RJ. Physiological basis: how NREM sleep components can promote and REM sleep components can suppress seizure discharge propagation. Clin Neurophysiol 2000; 111(Suppl 2):S9–18.

76. Swihart BJ, et al. Characterizing sleep structure using the hypnogram. J Clin Sleep Med 2008;4(4): 349–55.

77. Bazil CW. Seizure modulation by sleep and sleep state. Brain Res 2019;1703:13–7.

78. Vendrame M, et al. Effect of continuous positive airway pressure treatment on seizure control in patients with obstructive sleep apnea and epilepsy. Epilepsia 2011;52(11):e168–71.

79. Hollinger P, et al. Epilepsy and obstructive sleep apnea. Eur Neurol 2006;55(2):74–9.

80. Ng AK, Guan C. Impact of obstructive sleep apnea on sleep-wake stage ratio. Annu Int Conf IEEE Eng Med Biol Soc 2012;2012:4660–3.

81. Chervin RD, Shelgikar AV, Burns JW. Respiratory cycle-related EEG changes: response to CPAP. Sleep 2012;35(2):203–9.

82. Aldrich M, et al. Effects of continuous positive airway pressure on phasic events of REM sleep in patients with obstructive sleep apnea. Sleep 1989;12(5): 413–9.

83. Issa FG, Sullivan CE. The immediate effects of nasal continuous positive airway pressure treatment on sleep pattern in patients with obstructive sleep apnea syndrome. Electroencephalogr Clin Neurophysiol 1986;63(1):10–7.

84. Spalka J, et al. Morning headache as an obstructive sleep apnea-related symptom among sleep Clinic patients-A cross-section analysis. Brain Sci 2020; 10(1).

85. Smith MT, et al. The effects of sleep deprivation on pain inhibition and spontaneous pain in women. Sleep 2007;30(4):494–505.

86. Buse DC, et al. Sleep disorders among People with migraine: results from the chronic migraine epidemiology and outcomes (CaMEO) study. Headache 2019;59(1):32–45.

87. Ulfberg J, et al. Headache, snoring and sleep apnoea. J Neurol 1996;243(9):621–5.

88. Loh NK, et al. Do patients with obstructive sleep apnea wake up with headaches? Arch Intern Med 1999;159(15):1765–8.

89. Jensen R, et al. Is obstructive sleep apnea syndrome associated with headache? Acta Neurol Scand 2004;109(3):180–4.

90. Kristiansen HA, et al. Migraine and sleep apnea in the general population. J Headache Pain 2011; 12(1):55–61.

91. Schuh-Hofer S, et al. Increased serotonin transporter availability in the brainstem of migraineurs. J Neurol 2007;254(6):789–96.

92. Shoib S, Malik JA, Masoodi S. Depression as a Manifestation of obstructive sleep apnea. J Neurosci Rural Pract 2017;8(3):346–51.

93. Chiu YC, et al. Tension-type headache associated with obstructive sleep apnea: a nationwide population-based study. J Headache Pain 2015;16: 34.

94. Schain AJ, et al. Cortical spreading depression Closes Paravascular space and Impairs glymphatic Flow: implications for migraine headache. J Neurosci 2017;37(11):2904–15.

95. Johnson KG, Ziemba AM, Garb JL. Improvement in headaches with continuous positive airway pressure for obstructive sleep apnea: a retrospective analysis. Headache 2013;53(2):333–43.

96. Kallweit U, et al. Continuous positive airway pressure therapy is effective for migraines in sleep apnea syndrome. Neurology 2011;76(13):1189–91.

# Continuous Positive Airway Pressure Use for Obstructive Sleep Apnea in Pediatric Patients

Temitayo Oyegbile-Chidi, MD, PhD

## KEYWORDS

- Pediatric obstructive sleep apnea • CPAP • Genetic disorders • Obesity • Pediatric auto-CPAP
- Pediatric CPAP adherence

## KEY POINTS

- Pediatric obstructive sleep apnea is becoming more common, and practitioners are getting better at diagnosing and treating it. It is common in children with obesity, genetic disorders, neuromuscular disorders, and congenital malformations.
- After adenotonsillectomy, CPAP is one of the major modes of treatment. CPAP is traditionally initiated by titrating in the laboratory; however, auto-CPAP titration in the home environment is becoming more accepted as an option.
- When children are adherent to CPAP, there are significant benefits to treatment, which are short-term and long-term in nature.
- The short-term benefits include improved behavior, focus, attention, and improved sleep. The long-term benefits include improved cardiovascular and metabolic comorbidities.

## INTRODUCTION

Pediatric obstructive sleep apnea (OSA) is a sleep breathing disorder that is quickly becoming better recognized and diagnosed in the pediatric population.[1] This disorder differs significantly from that of adults by way of presentation, diagnosis criteria, treatment, and prognosis. Unlike its adult counterpart, pediatric OSA has been associated with multiple signs, symptoms, and comorbidities that are unique to the pediatric population including attention-deficit/hyperactivity disorder, nocturnal enuresis, craniofacial abnormalities, genetic syndromes, and neuromuscular disorders. These other signs, symptoms, syndromes, and comorbidities can frequently lead to delays in OSA diagnosis and treatment.[2]

The prevalence of this disorder is estimated at 5% to 6% and this prevalence is expected to rise with the worsening epidemic of childhood obesity.[3] In addition, the prevalence is significantly higher in children with certain disorders, such as trisomy 21 and mucolipidosis, where the prevalence is 50% to 100%.[1] The incidence ranges widely from newborns to teenagers and has two key peaks during the course of childhood. The first peak is in children ages 2 to 8 years, whereas the second peak is during adolescence.[4] Pediatric OSA can also lead to the development of notable neurobehavioral and medical sequela and long-term can increase the risk of cardiovascular and metabolic morbidity into early adulthood.[5–7] As a consequence, treatment of OSA in children is imperative.

Adenotonsillectomy (AT) is recommended as the first line of therapy, based on the American Academy of Pediatrics and the American Academy of Sleep Medicine guidelines. This surgical

Pediatric Neurology, Epilepsy and Sleep Medicine, Department of Neurology, UC Davis School of Medicine, MIND Institute, Center for Mind and Brain, University of California - Davis, 4860 Y Street, Sacramento, CA 95817, USA
E-mail address: oyegbilechidi@ucdavis.edu

Sleep Med Clin 17 (2022) 629–638
https://doi.org/10.1016/j.jsmc.2022.07.008
1556-407X/22/© 2022 Elsevier Inc. All rights reserved.

| Abbreviations | |
| --- | --- |
| CPAP | Continuous Postive Airway Pressure |
| OSA | Obstructive Sleep Apnea |
| AT | Adenotonsillectomy |
| NIV | Non-Invasive Ventilation |
| AHI | Apnea-Hypopnea Index |
| ENT | Ear, Nose & Throat |
| HFNC | High Flow Nasal Cannula |
| SDB | Sleep Disordered Breathing |
| REM | Rapid Eye Movement |

therapy has been shown to improve and sometimes completely alleviate the symptoms of OSA. AT can also improve behavior and quality of life.[8] A significant number of children require no further treatment/therapy; however, up to 73% of children continue to have residual symptoms of OSA postoperatively. These residual symptoms of OSA include unchanged or only slightly improved symptoms of snoring, neurobehavioral problems including hyperactivity and inattention, daytime sleepiness, and polysomnographic evidence of OSA after surgery. In addition, a significant number of children diagnosed with OSA are not ideal candidates for surgery. For these two groups of children (those with residual OSA and those who are not surgical candidates), the American Academy of Pediatrics and American Academy of Sleep Medicine recommend a trial of continuous positive airway pressure (CPAP).[9]

There is another subset of children in which OSA is more common and more severe, and is also associated with specific comorbidities, such as congenital craniofacial malformations (eg, Pierre Robin syndrome and Treacher Collins syndrome), complex craniofacial abnormalities, syndromic craniostenosis, metabolic/endocrinology disorders (eg, Prader-Willi syndrome), storage diseases (eg, mucopolysaccharidosis), genetic conditions (eg, trisomy 21). The disorders usually present with the so-called "complex pediatric OSA," where the airway obstruction is regarded as multifactorial and multileveled. Children with complex OSA are much more likely to experience persistent residual OSA after upper airway surgery and most often require CPAP after surgery.

There are no clear evidence-based pediatric guidelines for the duration and timing recommended for CPAP so current recommendations must be followed with caution because they are lifted from the adult guidelines literature. Currently, ideal CPAP use in children includes using the device during total and all physiologic sleep time, which may exceed 12 hours especially in infants and should include napping preferably. Minimal use follows the adult guidelines of 4 hours/night for at least 70% of nights over a 30-day period or 50% of sleep time.

Barriers to successful CPAP implementation in children include limited mask size options, limited titration capabilities in hospitals, and limited sleep specialists with pediatric expertise.[10] Furthermore, compliance with CPAP therapy is a major obstacle to treatment of OSA.[7] In addition, there are significant limitations associated with inferences made from CPAP-related research studies when extrapolated from the adult studies to the pediatric population because they fail to address pediatric-specific changes associated with growth, which can affect the risk of airway obstruction over time including changes in tone, airway caliber, and amount of lymphoid tissue.[3] Based on this information, frequent reevaluation of children on CPAP therapy is warranted to check and adjust the fitting of the CPAP equipment and the pressure settings. Furthermore, more research on CPAP use in children is necessary.

This article explores the use of CPAP in the pediatric population as a whole and within specific subsets of the pediatric population and also evaluates specific benefits, challenges, and potential future uses of CPAP within the pediatric OSA population.

## HISTORY OF CONTINUOUS POSITIVE AIRWAY PRESSURE USE IN CHILDREN

CPAP is increasingly being used as a treatment for OSA in children.[11] This therapy was first introduced into the pediatric population around 1984 to 1986.[10] In 1986, it was initially used in 10 children ages 3 to 11 years with a diagnosis of OSA. It was used to stent open the airway because these children had different types of congenital anomalies and developmental disorders.[12] By 1995, pediatric CPAP masks had increased in commercial availability[13] especially for large pediatric sleep disorders centers. At that time, CPAP was specifically used for OSA associated with obesity, craniofacial anomalies, trisomy 21, and residual OSA symptoms postsurgery. At the time, it was generally initiated during a CPAP titration study in a pediatric sleep laboratory at one of the large sleep centers for children. Over the next decade, sleep centers began to introduce a 2-week mask acclimatization period before the CPAP titration study to improve the chances of tolerating the mask and the CPAP setting during the overnight titration study. In 2021, improvements in CPAP use in the pediatric population have been limited but continue to advance. In addition, there is exciting research in the pipeline

**Table 1**
**Distribution of patients according to primary diagnosis**

| Nosologic Group | Patients (N = 68) n (%)[a] | OSA Plus Hypoventilation Syndrome n (%)[a] | Age at NIV Start, mo Median (IQR) |
|---|---|---|---|
| Congenital malformation/ genetic disorders | 34 (50) | 7 (10) | 42.5 (5–144) |
| Prader-Willi syndrome | 6 | 2 | 176 (158–187) |
| Pierre Robin syndrome | 5 | 0 | 1 (0–2) |
| Trisomy 21 | 5 | 2 | 12 (46–180) |
| Craniofacial malformation[b] | 10 | 0 | 40 (7–45) |
| Airway malacia | 5 | 0 | 13 (2–15) |
| Other | 3 | 3 | 60 (40–96) |
| Cerebral palsy | 9 (13) | 2 (3) | 168 (89–173) |
| Central nervous system tumor | 8 (12) | 1 (1.5) | 171 (94–180) |
| Inborn errors of metabolism | 6 (9) | 2 (3) | 59 (20–135) |
| Mucopolysaccharidosis | 5 | 2 | 59 (46–156) |
| Gaucher disease | 1 | 0 | 2 |
| Adenoid/tonsil hypertrophy | 3 (4) | 0 | 15 (12–31) |
| Obesity | 3 (4) | 0 | 166 (154–194) |
| Others | 5 (8) | 0 | 106 (85–110) |

*Abbreviations:* IQR, interquartile range; NIV, noninvasive ventilation.
[a] All percentages refer to the total number of patients (N = 68).
[b] Including choanal atresia, craniosynostosis, pycnodysostosis, achondroplasia, CHARGE syndrome.
Girbal et al. Non-invasive ventilation in complex obstructive sleep apnea – A 15-year experience of a pediatric tertiary center, Revista Portuguesa de Pneumologia (English Edition), 20 (3), 2014, 146-151, https://doi.org/10.1016/j.rppnen.2014.05.001.

and potential auto-CPAP options on the horizon, which is discussed further in this article.

## DISORDERS ASSOCIATED WITH COMPLEX OBSTRUCTIVE SLEEP APNEA REQUIRING EARLY/FIRST-LINE CONTINUOUS POSITIVE AIRWAY PRESSURE TREATMENT

There is a group of disorders and syndromes associated with pediatric OSA where CPAP is often considered the first-line treatment of choice (**Table 1**).[14] These children tend to experience significant upper and sometimes lower airway obstruction including those with tracheobronchomalacia or bronchopulmonary dysplasia.[11] Increased elasticity of the soft tissues in the upper and lower airway lumen may play a significant role in the clinician's choice as to whether to start CPAP as a first-line treatment.[15] Pediatric laryngomalacia is a disorder where up to 78% of patients develop OSA. Treatment, possibly initially with surgical intervention, and subsequently certainly with CPAP is crucial to long-term care.[16]

Infants with craniofacial malformations, such as Pierre Robin syndrome, Goldenhar syndrome, trisomy 21, Treacher Collins syndrome, velocardiofacial syndrome, and cleft lip and palate, require close monitoring because of the concern of OSA development and recurrence over time, which is especially taxing and can quickly lead to deterioration of health.[17] Children with Schwartz-Jampel syndrome can end up with severe OSA and often require surgical intervention, such as rapid maxillary expansion to improve the benefits of CPAP therapy, as seen in **Fig. 1**.[18]

Pediatric OSA should also be considered in certain genetic disorders including DiGeorge syndrome (22q11.2 syndrome), which is associated with velopharyngeal insufficiency, and Prader-Willi syndrome and trisomy 21, which are associated with significant hypotonia. Several neuromuscular disorders also require CPAP as first-line treatment. These syndromes frequently require initial surgical treatment of the velopharyngeal insufficiency/airway obstruction and postsurgical CPAP for the residual moderate to severe OSA.[19–21] Children with genetic disorders and OSA often have behavioral and developmental delays, which can lead to difficulty initiating and implementing CPAP postsurgery for residual OSA. Such disorders as Prader-Willi are also associated with excessive daytime sleepiness and extreme weight

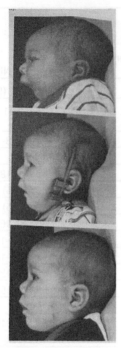

**Fig. 1.** Surgical interventions over time that improve CPAP usefulness (sleep secrets).

gain. Weight loss is often considered a therapeutic option in this population; however, this can take time and is variable as the child grows and matures. Therefore, CPAP remains a mainstay of therapy in these subpopulations of children with persistent (residual) OSA.

Obesity is rapidly becoming the disorder most commonly associated with pediatric OSA.[5] Depending on the country, prevalence levels of obesity are 7% to 22% and this disorder can adversely affect multiple organ systems. As such, the prevalence of pediatric OSA in obese children is 21% to 40%. Neurocognitive and behavioral problems, cardiovascular abnormalities (increased nocturnal systolic blood pressure, sustained diurnal hypertension, and left ventricular changes), and endothelial and metabolic dysfunction are frequent consequences of OSA, which are further worsened by the combination of obesity and OSA. Specifically, the combination of obesity and OSA in children can lead to significant metabolic comorbidities including dyslipidemia, insulin resistance, metabolic syndrome, and cardiovascular morbidity, which can lead to significant metabolic and physiologic problems into adulthood.[22]

## CONTINUOUS POSITIVE AIRWAY PRESSURE TITRATION

The use of CPAP to treat OSA in children has been increasing over the years.[23] In general, initiation of

CPAP is achieved in a pediatric sleep laboratory where a CPAP titration study is performed overnight. Two weeks before the CPAP titration study night, the child undergoes mask acclimatization. CPAP has been shown to be efficacious in improving polysomnogram parameters including apnea-hypoxia index (AHI), respiratory effort–related arousals, and patient and caregiver daytime sleepiness.[10] CPAP is not yet approved by the Food and Drug Administration for use in children weighing less than 30 kg; however, it is frequently used in a wide range of ages from newborns to adolescent years, especially in the setting of complex OSA and associated comorbidities. Fitting of the CPAP equipment and adjustment of the pressure settings must be individualized for each child and should be managed by health care professionals with expertise in the management of pediatric sleep patients.[24] A recently published algorithm can assist in correctly assessing the CPAP titration plan (**Fig. 2**).[11] It is important to ensure the device settings correspond with prescribed settings. Infant CPAP devices often underestimate the real use of the device. Continuous monitoring of CPAP equipment includes frequent periodic polysomnogram evaluation especially if the child's symptoms change, significant growth/puberty occur, and/or if the body mass index increases or decreases.[9] Unlike in adult studies, CPAP requirements in children rapidly change with growth. Up to a quarter of children started on CPAP need an adjustment within 3 months.[9,13]

CPAP therapy efficacy findings are heterogeneous within the pediatric population.[25] In infants, data on the effectiveness of CPAP use are sparse, even though it can be standard of therapy for treatment of complex OSA.[26] Compared with school-aged children ages 5 to 10 years of age, CPAP in infants less than 6 months of age is highly effective in treating OSA and well-tolerated, especially when used along with other treatment options, such as surgery.[26] In addition to being efficacious, CPAP is also considered safe and fairly well-tolerated overall in children and adolescents.[13]

## CONTINUOUS POSITIVE AIRWAY PRESSURE AUTOTITRATION

In general, CPAP titration studies performed overnight in the sleep laboratory have been the standard of care to determine precise therapeutic CPAP settings for children. Currently, it is considered the gold standard for CPAP initiation and monitoring in children with OSA. CPAP autotitration is rarely considered and is usually reserved for older children.[6,27] Recent advancements in CPAP technology may increase the chances of young children

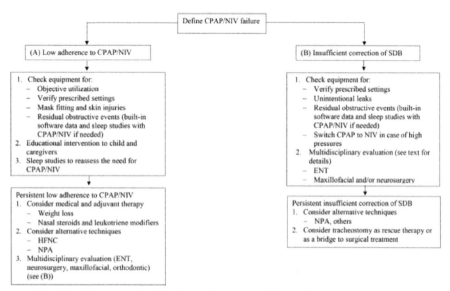

**Fig. 2.** Proposed algorithm for CPAP titration, low adherence, and low adherence persistence. ENT, ear, nose, and throat; HFNC, high-flow nasal cannula; NIV, noninvasive ventilation; NPA, nasopharyngeal airway; SDB, sleep-disordered breathing. (*From* Amaddeo et al., 2020.)

successfully initiating CPAP (auto-CPAP) in the home environment. Furthermore, these auto-CPAP devices enable an approach where monitoring is frequently and seamlessly continued after successful CPAP commencement.[28]

There are several disadvantages to having a child spend the night in sleep laboratory including discomfort, cost, and inability to sleep in a new environment, which can lead to delays in achieving therapeutic CPAP settings. Furthermore, the specific mechanics of the pediatric airflow (smaller airway sizes, faster respiratory rates, and other respiratory parameters) make children and pediatric OSA unique such that individualizing CPAP settings is more desirable to optimize care. As such, CPAP autotitration may be advantageous because it may function as a cost-effective and economical approach to treating OSA while initiating and monitoring treatment efficaciously at limited cost to the caregiver and reduced discomfort to the child. Autotitrating CPAP and using remote modem monitoring over time can prove to be useful compared with fixed pressure CPAP alone. Although not perfectly equivalent, auto-CPAP has been shown to deliver treatment pressures that are fairly similar to the gold standard of manual CPAP titration in the laboratory.[28]

It is also important to note that fixed CPAP titration pressure that is set in the laboratory is set high enough to eliminate all obstructive events during the night. Often, a child may not need such a high pressure throughout the night because CPAP needs may change depending on sleep stage (eg, REM, N3 deep sleep) and sleep position (eg, supine, lateral, prone). Auto-CPAP is more flexible so that the mean pressure is an average of the required pressures titrated throughout the night to successfully eliminate all/most obstructive events and is usually lower than the fixed titration pressure derived from CPAP titration studies in the laboratory. Some studies have found that auto-CPAP settings through the night tend to be adequate to treat and essentially eliminate most obstructive events, whereas others have found that a residual but significant number of apnea and hypopnea events may remain.[6,29] As the CPAP technology continues to advance and algorithms get more detailed/focused to adequately and accurately address all the obstructive events in children with OSA overnight, the usefulness of auto-CPAP in childhood OSA will most likely increase.

There are, however, some major limitations currently to using auto-CPAP to treat pediatric OSA. Each CPAP manufacturer uses a unique proprietary algorithm to determine appropriate CPAP for each CPAP device type. These algorithms are rarely tested on children before launch and thus may not be optimized for use in children with OSA. In addition, different auto-CPAP machine types respond differently to the same respiratory events. Given the differences in pediatric airway mechanics, the CPAP machine type may be more likely to provide an inappropriate/inaccurate response for specific respiratory obstructive events.[6,23] In addition, the acceptable residual AHI level differs between adults with OSA and children with OSA (ie, AHI <5/hour in adults vs AHI <1/hour in children) and may lead to a delay in the response of the device to respiratory events because most auto-CPAP devices are set to change settings with an AHI >5 hour (adult settings) instead of an AHI greater than 1/hour (child settings).

Overall, pediatric auto-CPAP is a treatment option that is yet to be fully embraced within the pediatric sleep specialist community but this is likely to change in the future. One of the major reasons for the community's current reticence is the paucity of research available on the use of auto-CPAP in children. For now, the general recommendations suggest using a traditional CPAP titration study in the laboratory to initiate CPAP, because this is the gold standard,[27] and subsequently use of an auto-CPAP device for frequent assessment to monitor CPAP settings in the outpatient clinic between in-laboratory PSG evaluations.

## BENEFITS OF CONTINUOUS POSITIVE AIRWAY PRESSURE

Efficacy CPAP research in children and young adolescents is limited; however, CPAP seems to be beneficial overall. Children with OSA using CPAP seem to have significant relief of symptoms of OSA and seem to have improvement in the physical, emotional, and behavioral complications, especially when used consistently.[30] After 6 months of CPAP treatment, systolic blood pressure can significantly decrease.[31] In children with cerebral palsy, CPAP treatment of OSA improved the quality of life.[32] Children with epilepsy and OSA using CPAP had improvement in seizure control.[33] In obese children, after using CPAP for 1 year to treat OSA, C-reactive protein, high-density lipoprotein, and low-density lipoprotein were significantly improved.[5,22] CPAP use is also associated with improvement in attention, working memory, and depression in children with OSA.[34] A small study of nine children with OSA and nonalcoholic fatty liver disease monitored CPAP use and metabolic markers for a total of 3 months. With CPAP treatment, participants had increased duration of sleep with improvement of their sleep apnea severity. Severity of liver injury, markers of metabolic syndrome, and reduced oxidative stress also improved significantly.[35] In another small study evaluating obese children with OSA, leptin levels improved significantly after CPAP treatment.[36] Even with low adherence of CPAP use, CPAP benefits are still evident. With mean nightly usage of only 3 hours per night, there were significant improvements after 3 months in the AHI and neurobehavioral assessments of attention deficits,

sleepiness, and behavior. Overall, the limited evidence available indicates that CPAP therapy is beneficial for sleep parameters, daytime symptoms, quality of life, and metabolic parameters.

## CONTINUOUS POSITIVE AIRWAY PRESSURE ADHERENCE

As seen in adults, CPAP adherence levels in children with OSA can be poor, and similar to that of several other pediatric chronic illness treatments. These poor adherence levels in children and adolescents with OSA often begin soon after CPAP commencement, averaging 3.35 hours per night.[30,37] In addition, the prevalence of CPAP refusal is high at 25% to 50%.[24] One study showed that CPAP use was the highest during the first week of commencement at 79% of nights and then declined over time in a group of children with OSA.[38] By the end of the first month, CPAP use had decreased to 65% of nights and was 57% of nights by the end of the 3-month period. Nightly use of CPAP also declined from 3.5 hours nightly by the end of the first week of CPAP commencement to 2.8 hours nightly at the end of the third month.

Several factors contribute to the level of CPAP adoption and adherence. Female children are more likely to have good adherence compared with male children. This pattern is also seen in other chronic pediatric illnesses. Parental behavioral management strategies, monitoring, and differing expectations for boys and girls may explain this pattern. Socioeconomic status and increased body mass index (obesity) do not seem to play a significant role in CPAP adherence; however, older age of the child may be associated with lower CPAP adherence.[37] Maternal education is the one factor that has been shown consistently to be associated with increased CPAP adherence. Parental motivation and perception of CPAP benefit are also some important determinants of CPAP adherence.[10]

Children with OSA and disabilities, especially intellectual disabilities, are a unique subset of children with OSA because their CPAP adherence and compliance levels are often high even though one may presume otherwise. In several studies evaluating children with OSA and trisomy 21, CPAP adherence was high.[39,40] These children were monitored over a 2-year period and CPAP adherence started at 50% to 57% and was 39% to 67% 2 years later. On average, nightly use was greater than 4 hours. This excellent adherence that persists over a prolonged period of time may be caused by increased dependence on caregivers, increased parental perception of the need for CPAP, and perhaps a decreased ability to remove the mask at night.

Nasal complaints also contribute to poor CPAP adherence and are improved by treating with topical nasal steroids and addition of humidification to the CPAP. In one study, 64 children with OSA received CPAP and 26% were intolerant of initial CPAP therapy. After home mask acclimatization, change in mask size, skin cream use, and addition of passive humidification, 37% of these children eventually accepted and adhered to CPAP therapy.[41] CPAP treatment post-AT may also be associated with poorer adherence compared with CPAP treatment as first-line therapy.[42] In these situations, increased caregiver support and switching to bilevel support can improve CPAP adherence.[43] CPAP adherence improves when another family member is also concurrently using CPAP.

Several studies have found that outpatient initiation of CPAP therapy (auto-CPAP) may be associated with a higher level of adherence.[27] Using the home environment as the setting to initiate CPAP can also lead to more successful implementation and adherence. One study assessing the use of auto-CPAP versus fixed CPAP pressure showed a trend toward longer duration of CPAP use per day in those children younger than age 13 who used auto-CPAP compared with control subjects who used fixed CPAP.[28] However, other research groups suggest that starting CPAP therapy in the home (auto-CPAP) may not make much difference to CPAP adherence.[44] Another study showed that discrepancies between in-laboratory fixed CPAP recommendations and at-home auto-CPAP device settings can result in discomfort and early reduced CPAP adherence. Ensuring similarity between the in-laboratory CPAP titration study setting and the home auto-CPAP settings is a key to accomplishing early adherence of CPAP treatment and reduction of discomfort.[23,29] Overall, troubleshooting and adjusting CPAP settings as needed can help improve adherence to CPAP that may initially have been poorly tolerated.

Studies have shown that CPAP adherence is certainly cost-effective from a financial standpoint, a health care utilization standpoint, and for quality of life.[45] It is also important from a cognitive and behavioral standpoint because attention span, sleepiness, behavior problems, caregiver quality of life, and child quality of life are significantly improved.[44,46] CPAP adherence in children can certainly be improved with desensitization measures and behavioral interventions along with frequent home visits and periodic revaluations using follow-up sleep studies in the laboratory.[44]

These desensitization measures and behavioral interventions have been recommended to improve CPAP adherence including parent training and modeling. Behavioral training has been proven to be efficacious, leading to continued adherence up to 9 months later.[46] Shared decision-making tools could also potentially improve CPAP adherence and health outcomes.[47] Among families of children with OSA who may not be surgical candidates, shared decision-making tools have been used to counsel on the best treatment options. Using this strategy, families were more likely to agree to and adhere to CPAP treatment with improved health outcomes long-term.[47] Overall, supportive interventions, educational interventions, and behavioral therapy for child and caregiver are crucial for adequate CPAP adherence in children. Age-adjusted and development-adjusted interventions must match the child's needs to ensure successful and cost-effective CPAP implementation.

## EFFICACY OF CONTINUOUS POSITIVE AIRWAY PRESSURE VERSUS OTHER OBSTRUCTIVE SLEEP APNEA TREATMENT OPTIONS

Pediatric OSA can either be treated using AT or CPAP as the first-line treatment. Evidence indicates that AT and CPAP may be equally efficacious, especially in children with trisomy 21 or mucolipidosis who have mild to moderate OSA.[1,48] CPAP may be more effective than AT in moderate to severe complex OSA associated with myelomeningocele.[49] CPAP tends to show immediate sustained improvement, whereas AT tends to show a more gradual improvement.[1] Furthermore, AT is more frequently associated with weight gain compared with CPAP.[37]

To improve CPAP adherence, sleep specialists often recommend a trial bilevel positive airway pressure therapy. Indeed, bilevel positive airway pressure shows higher adherence levels compared with CPAP at a 1-year follow-up, especially in nonobese patients.[44,50] However, no differences were noted in efficiency between CPAP and bilevel positive airway pressure.

In the setting of CPAP failure, along with noncompliance and/or nontolerance of CPAP, high-flow nasal cannula is considered as an option.[51] There is limited evidence of the efficacy comparisons between CPAP and high-flow nasal cannula.

## SIDE EFFECTS OF CONTINUOUS POSITIVE AIRWAY PRESSURE

As with adults on CPAP, children using CPAP frequently experience nasal bridge sores from masks, abdominal distention, mouth and nasal/

pharyngeal dryness, nasal congestion, rhinorrhea, epistaxis, eye irritation, and overall discomfort from air leaks, especially in the setting of a poorly fitting mask.[13,24,44] These side effects can affect at least 30% of children after 5 months of use.[52] Claustrophobia and social anxiety may also develop from CPAP therapy. Depending on developmental age, very young children on CPAP can experience midface flattening, maxillary retrusion, counter-clockwise rotation of the palatal plane, and upper incisor flaring from long-standing pressure of the mask on the face.[3] The mask pressure can significantly affect growing facial features in children with OSA on CPAP and must be carefully monitored with digital photography.

## DISCONTINUATION OF CONTINUOUS POSITIVE AIRWAY PRESSURE

Unlike in adults, children with OSA can outgrow the diagnosis of pediatric OSA as they develop. Some children can experience full resolution of their OSA without any obvious intervention apart from the CPAP. Others can show improvement in their body mass index; however, this is less likely to completely resolve the OSA. Surgical airway intervention can also significantly assist in improving OSA. As a consequence, CPAP continuation monitoring by the clinician is imperative. Evidence suggests that monitoring should be considered at least annually, and more frequently, if clinically indicated. CPAP therapy may successfully be discontinued after about 1 year of use.[3] More specifically, children with minimal-mild residual OSA after a year are considered for discontinuation with close monitoring.

## FUTURE OF CONTINUOUS POSITIVE AIRWAY PRESSURE USE IN CHILDREN

In the next decade, it is likely auto-CPAP will be used more widely among pediatric sleep specialists because overnight manual titration is costly, time consuming, resource intense, and not available in all settings. CPAP predictive equations are frequently used in adults. In the last couple years, researchers have begun to evaluate predictive optimal equations to determine the best CPAP settings for children with OSA based on pediatric airway and respiratory mechanics.[53] The applicability needs to be tested within different age ranges to determine usefulness, validity, and reliability. These findings are necessary to advance auto-CPAP use in children with OSA. Furthermore, to appropriately determine those who may or may not benefit from behavioral therapy and supportive interventions for improved CPAP adherence,

researchers are beginning to use hierarchical clustering.[25,54] When clustered by CPAP tolerance and use over time, obesity, CPAP setting, developmental delay, and prior AT played a role. As a result, this analytical approach may provide some insight into how to optimize CPAP therapy.[25] Over the next decade, these findings and more may become helpful in improving CPAP therapy and compliance.

## DISCLOSURE

The project described was also supported by the National Center for Advancing Translational Sciences, National Institutes of Health, through grant number UL1 TR001860 and linked award KL2 TR001859. The content is solely the responsibility of the authors and does not necessarily represent the official views of the NIH.

## REFERENCES

1. Sudarsan SS, Paramasivan VK, Arumugam SV, et al. Comparison of treatment modalities in syndromic children with obstructive sleep apnea: a randomized cohort study. Int J Pediatr Otorhinolaryngol 2014; 78(9):1526–33.
2. Alsubie HS, BaHammam AS. Obstructive sleep apnoea: children are not little adults. Paediatr Respir Rev 2017;21:72–9.
3. King Z, Josee-Leclerc M, Wales P, et al. Can CPAP therapy in pediatric OSA ever be stopped? J Clin Sleep Med 2019;15(11):1609–12.
4. Katz ES, D'Ambrosio CM. Pathophysiology of pediatric obstructive sleep apnea. Proc Am Thorac Soc 2008;5(2):253–62.
5. Alonso-Álvarez ML, Terán-Santos J, Gonzalez Martinez M, et al, Spanish Sleep Network. Metabolic biomarkers in community obese children: effect of obstructive sleep apnea and its treatment. Sleep Med 2017;37:1–9.
6. Khaytin I, Tapia IE, Xanthopoulos MS, et al. Auto-titrating CPAP for the treatment of obstructive sleep apnea in children. J Clin Sleep Med 2020;16(6):871–8.
7. Whitla L, Lennon P. Non-surgical management of obstructive sleep apnoea: a review. Paediatrics Int Child Health 2017;37(1):1–5.
8. Marcus CL, Moore RH, Rosen CL, et al, Childhood Adenotonsillectomy Trial (CHAT). A randomized trial of adenotonsillectomy for childhood sleep apnea. N Engl J Med 2013;368(25):2366–76.
9. Marcus CL, Brooks LJ, Draper KA, et al, American Academy of Pediatrics. Diagnosis and management of childhood obstructive sleep apnea syndrome. Pediatrics 2012;130(3):e714–55.
10. Wang JJ, Imamura T, Lee J, et al. Continuous positive airway pressure for obstructive sleep apnea in children. Can Fam Physician 2021;67(1):21–3.

11. Amaddeo A, Khirani S, Griffon L, et al. Non-invasive ventilation and CPAP failure in children and indications for invasive ventilation. Front Pediatr 2020;8: 544921.

12. Guilleminault C, Nino-Murcia G, Heldt G, et al. Alternative treatment to tracheostomy in obstructive sleep apnea syndrome: nasal continuous positive airway pressure in young children. Pediatrics 1986; 78(5):797–802.

13. Marcus CL, Ward SL, Mallory GB, et al. Use of nasal continuous positive airway pressure as treatment of childhood obstructive sleep apnea. J Pediatr 1995; 127(1):88–94.

14. Girbal C, Gonçalves C, Nunes T, Ferreira R, Pereira L, Saianda A, Bandeira T. Non-invasive ventilation in complex obstructive sleep apnea–a 15-year experience of a pediatric tertiary center. Rev Port Pneumol 2014 May-Jun;20(3):146–51. https://doi.org/10.1016/j.rppneu.2013.08.001. PMID: 24525398.

15. Subramaniam DR, Mylavarapu G, McConnell K, et al. Upper airway elasticity estimation in pediatric down syndrome sleep apnea patients using collapsible tube theory. Ann Biomed Eng 2016;44(5): 1538–52.

16. Verkest V, Verhulst S, Van Hoorenbeeck K, et al. Prevalence of obstructive sleep apnea in children with laryngomalacia and value of polysomnography in treatment decisions. Int J Pediatr Otorhinolaryngol 2020;137:110255.

17. Amaddeo A, Griffon L, Fauroux B. Using continuous nasal airway pressure in infants with craniofacial malformations. Semin Fetal Neonatal Med 2021; 101284. https://doi.org/10.1016/j.siny.2021.101284.

18. Peanchitlertkajorn S, Assawakawintip T, Pibulniyom M, et al. Successful treatment of a child with Schwartz-Jampel syndrome using rapid maxillary expansion and CPAP. J Clin Sleep Med 2021;17(3):601–4.

19. Crockett DJ, Goudy SL, Chinnadurai S, et al. Obstructive sleep apnea syndrome in children with 22q11.2 deletion syndrome after operative intervention for velopharyngeal insufficiency. Front Pediatr 2014;2:84.

20. Gillett ES, Perez IA. Disorders of sleep and ventilatory control in Prader-Willi syndrome. Diseases 2016;4(3):23.

21. Waters KA, Castro C, Chawla J. The spectrum of obstructive sleep apnea in infants and children with Down syndrome. Int J Pediatr Otorhinolaryngol 2020;129:109763.

22. Amini Z, Kotagal S, Lohse C, et al. Effect of obstructive sleep apnea treatment on lipids in obese children. Children 2017;4(6):44.

23. Mihai R, Ellis K, Davey MJ, et al. Interpreting CPAP device respiratory indices in children. J Clin Sleep Med 2020;16(10):1655–61.

24. Rana M, August J, Levi J, et al. Alternative approaches to adenotonsillectomy and continuous positive airway pressure (CPAP) for the management of pediatric obstructive sleep apnea (OSA): a review. Sleep Disord 2020;7987208. https://doi.org/10.1155/2020/7987208.

25. Weiss MR, Allen ML, Landeo-Gutierrez JS, et al. Defining the patterns of PAP adherence in pediatric obstructive sleep apnea: a clustering analysis using real-world data. J Clin Sleep Med 2021;17(5): 1005–13.

26. Cielo CM, Hernandez P, Ciampaglia AM, et al. Positive airway pressure for the treatment of OSA in infants. Chest 2021;159(2):810–7.

27. Amaddeo A, Frapin A, Touil S, et al. Outpatient initiation of long-term continuous positive airway pressure in children. Pediatr Pulmonol 2018;53(10): 1422–8.

28. Mulholland A, Mihai R, Ellis K, et al. Paediatric CPAP in the digital age. Sleep Med 2021;84:352–5.

29. Mihai R, Vandeleur M, Pecoraro S, et al. Autotitrating CPAP as a tool for CPAP initiation for children. J Clin Sleep Med 2017;13(5):713–9.

30. Simon SL, Duncan CL, Janicke DM, et al. Barriers to treatment of paediatric obstructive sleep apnoea: development of the adherence barriers to continuous positive airway pressure (CPAP) questionnaire. Sleep Med 2012;13(2):172–7.

31. DelRosso LM, King J, Ferri R. Systolic blood pressure elevation in children with obstructive sleep apnea is improved with positive airway pressure use. J Pediatr 2018;195:102–7.e1.

32. Hsiao KH, Nixon GM. The effect of treatment of obstructive sleep apnea on quality of life in children with cerebral palsy. Res Dev Disabil 2008;29(2): 133–40.

33. Malow BA, Weatherwax KJ, Chervin RD, et al. Identification and treatment of obstructive sleep apnea in adults and children with epilepsy: a prospective pilot study. Sleep Med 2003;4(6):509–15.

34. Hobzova M, Hubackova L, Vanek J, et al. Cognitive function and depressivity before and after CPAP treatment in obstructive sleep apnea patients. Neuro Endocrinol Lett 2017;38(3):145–53.

35. Sundaram SS, Halbower AC, Klawitter J, et al. Treating obstructive sleep apnea and chronic intermittent hypoxia improves the severity of nonalcoholic fatty liver disease in children. J Pediatr 2018;198:67–75.e1.

36. Nakra N, Bhargava S, Dzuira J, et al. Sleep-disordered breathing in children with metabolic syndrome: the role of leptin and sympathetic nervous system activity and the effect of continuous positive airway pressure. Pediatrics 2008;122(3):e634–42.

37. Verhulst S. Long term continuous positive airway pressure and non-invasive ventilation in obstructive sleep apnea in children with obesity and down syndrome. Front Pediatr 2020;8:534.

38. Puri P, Ross KR, Mehra R, et al. Pediatric positive airway pressure adherence in obstructive sleep

apnea enhanced by family member positive airway pressure usage. J Clin Sleep Med 2016;12(7): 959–63.

39. Dudoignon B, Amaddeo A, Frapin A, et al. Obstructive sleep apnea in Down syndrome: benefits of surgery and noninvasive respiratory support. Am J Med Genet A 2017;173(8):2074–80.

40. Trucco F, Chatwin M, Semple T, et al. Sleep disordered breathing and ventilatory support in children with Down syndrome. Pediatr Pulmonol 2018; 53(10):1414–21.

41. Massa F, Gonsalez S, Laverty A, et al. The use of nasal continuous positive airway pressure to treat obstructive sleep apnoea. Arch Dis Child 2002; 87(5):438–43.

42. Pomerantz J. Management of persistent obstructive sleep apnea after adenotonsillectomy. Pediatr Ann 2016;45(5):e180–3.

43. Sawunyavisuth B, Ngamjarus C, Sawanyawisuth K. Any effective intervention to improve CPAP adherence in children with obstructive sleep apnea: a systematic review. Glob Pediatr Health 2021;8. 2333794X211019884.

44. Gozal D, Tan H-L, Kheirandish-Gozal L. Treatment of obstructive sleep apnea in children: handling the unknown with precision. J Clin Med 2020;9(3):888.

45. Hawkins SMM, Jensen EL, Simon SL, et al. Correlates of pediatric CPAP adherence. J Clin Sleep Med 2016;12(6):879–84.

46. Rains JC. Treatment of obstructive sleep apnea in pediatric patients. Behavioral intervention for compliance with nasal continuous positive airway pressure. Clin Pediatr 1995;34(10):535–41.

47. Bergeron M, Duggins A, Chini B, et al. Clinical outcomes after shared decision-making tools with families of children with obstructive sleep apnea without tonsillar hypertrophy. Laryngoscope 2019;129(11): 2646–51.

48. Venekamp RP, Hearne BJ, Chandrasekharan D, et al. Tonsillectomy or adenotonsillectomy versus non-surgical management for obstructive sleep-disordered breathing in children. Cochrane Database Syst Rev 2015;10:CD011165.

49. Kirk VG, Morielli A, Gozal D, et al. Treatment of sleep-disordered breathing in children with myelomeningocele. Pediatr Pulmonol 2000;30(6):445–52.

50. Machaalani R, Evans CA, Waters KA. Objective adherence to positive airway pressure therapy in an Australian paediatric cohort. Sleep Breath 2016; 20(4):1327–36.

51. Amaddeo A, Khirani S, Frapin A, et al. High-flow nasal cannula for children not compliant with continuous positive airway pressure. Sleep Med 2019;63: 24–8.

52. Marcus CL, Rosen G, Davidson Ward SL, et al. Adherence to and effectiveness of positive airway pressure therapy in children with obstructive sleep apnea. Pediatrics 2006;117(3). https://doi.org/10. 1542/peds.2005-1634.

53. Chong J, Bajpai R, Teoh OH, et al. Predictive equation for optimal continuous positive airway pressure in children with obstructive sleep apnoea. ERJ Open Res 2020;6(2). 00312–02019.

54. Tabone L, Caillaud C, Amaddeo A, et al. Sleep-disordered breathing in children with mucolipidosis. Am J Med Genet A 2019;179(7):1196–204.

# The Relationship Between Epilepsy, Obstructive Sleep Apnea, and Treatment Outcome

Nitin K. Sethi, MD, MBBS

## KEYWORDS

- Epilepsy • Sleep • Sleep apnea • Obstructive sleep apnea • Sleep disordered breathing
- Vagus nerve stimulator

## KEY POINTS

- A complex bidirectional relationship exists between epilepsy and obstructive sleep apnea (OSA).
- The coexistence of the 2 conditions adversely affects seizure control, OSA severity, and quality of life.
- Effective continuous positive airway pressure therapy in epilepsy patients with OSA may also result in improved seizure control.

## BACKGROUND

Epilepsy is one of the most common neurologic conditions with a reported prevalence of more than 50 million people worldwide.[1] As per the International League Against Epilepsy (ILAE), a person is considered to have epilepsy if they meet any of the following conditions—at least 2 unprovoked (or reflex) seizures occurring greater than 24 hours apart, one unprovoked (or reflex) seizure and a probability of further seizures similar to the general recurrence risk (at least 60%) after 2 unprovoked seizures occurring over the next 10 years, and lastly if a diagnosis of an epilepsy syndrome is established. Epilepsy is considered resolved for an individual who had an age-dependent epilepsy syndrome but has remained seizure free for the past 10 years and off antiseizure medication for the last 5 years.[2] Epilepsy is a heterogenous disease and can be of many types. In 2017, the ILAE updated the classification of epilepsies to consider the results of electroencephalography (EEG), neuroimaging studies, and underlying cause of the epilepsy.[3] There are now well-defined epilepsy syndromes that occur in the pediatric and adult population.[4] The global burden of epilepsy is enormous, and 80% of people with epilepsy live in low- and middle-income countries.[5] The current prevalence of epilepsy in the United States is thought to be around 2.2 million people or 7.1 for every 1000 people.[6] The treatment of epilepsy has also evolved over the years. Nowadays, there are many treatment options for epilepsy available including multiple antiseizure medications with different mechanisms of action, neuromodulation devices, and stimulators such as Vagus Nerve Stimulator (VNS), Responsive Neurostimulator (RNS), Deep Brain Stimulator (DBS), and resective epilepsy surgery.[7]

Obstructive sleep apnea (OSA) syndrome defined as apnea-hypopnea index (AHI) of 5 or greater is common with a reported mean prevalence of 22% (range, 9%–37%) in men and 17% (range, 4%–50%) in women.[8] It commonly occurs in people who are obese, with a large neck

Author contributions: N.K. Sethi conceived, drafted, and revised the manuscript.
Study funding: no targeted funding reported.
Data sharing statement: the author has no additional data to share.
Department of Neurology, New York-Presbyterian Hospital, Weill Cornell Medical Center, 525 East 68th Street, New York, NY 10065, USA
E-mail address: sethinitinmd@hotmail.com

diameter or congenitally narrow oropharynx causing mechanical airflow obstruction during sleep.[9]

With such an enormous global burden of both diseases, coexistence of epilepsy and OSA is common. The understanding of the complex bidirectional relationship between the 2 conditions and how the presence of one affects the other continues to evolve. To understand the relationship between epilepsy and OSA, one needs to first dwell into the intricate relationship between epilepsy and sleep.

## RELATIONSHIP BETWEEN EPILEPSY AND SLEEP

A complex bidirectional relationship exists between epilepsy and sleep. Some patients with epilepsy have both daytime and nocturnal seizures, whereas in others, seizures exclusively occur during sleep confirming the complex relationship between seizures and an individual's circadian pattern. It is also well recognized that seizures occur more commonly in some stages of sleep as compared with others. Herman and colleagues studied 613 seizures in 133 patients. Forty-three percent (264 of 613) of all partial seizures began during sleep. Nocturnal seizures began during stages N1 (23%) and N2 (68%) but were rare in slow-wave sleep (N3); no seizures were documented during rapid eye movement (REM) sleep in their cohort.[10] REM sleep is characterized by desynchronization of EEG, and hence seizure threshold is significantly higher in REM as compared with non-REM sleep.[11]

Secondary generalization of seizures has been noted to occur during sleep. In Herman and colleagues' study temporal lobe complex partial seizures are more likely to secondarily generalize during sleep (31%) than during wakefulness (15%), whereas frontal lobe seizures were less likely to secondarily generalize during sleep (10% vs 26%; $P < .005$).[10] Frontal lobe seizures tend to be nocturnal (highest incidence between 12 AM and 12 PM), whereas seizures originating from the temporal lobe are frequently diurnal (most frequent between 12 PM and 12 AM).[12]

Patients with autosomal dominant nocturnal frontal lobe epilepsy frequently have nocturnal seizures lasting from a few seconds to a few minutes and which tend to cluster. The clinical semiology ranges from bizarre hyperkinetic movements such as bicycling movements of the legs to abrupt arousals out of sleep (confusional arousals) without any associated motor phenomenology. The multiple seizures cause disruption of sleep architecture and are frequently initially misdiagnosed as parasomnias.[13] Other epilepsy syndromes such as Landau-Kleffner syndrome, generalized tonic-clonic seizures on waking, and continuous spike and wave during slow-wave sleep share a complex and yet to be fully elucidated relationship with sleep.[14,15]

Some epilepsy syndromes exhibit particularly strong circadian patterns. In patients with benign partial epilepsy with centrotemporal spikes and Panayiotopoulos syndrome, seizures usually emerge from sleep.[16] Patients with juvenile myoclonic epilepsy (JME) report more myoclonic jerks after a night of poor sleep. Sleep deprivation is a potent seizure-activating factor in these patients, and many patients with JME come to medical attention after suffering a generalized tonic-clonic convulsion following a night of sleep deprivation.[17]

Along with photic stimulation and hyperventilation, sleep deprivation remains a provocative measure in customary practice in EEG laboratories to increase the likelihood of capturing and characterizing seizures. Whether sleep deprivation alone though is sufficient to provoke a seizure remains unclear. It is the coming together of multiple factors such as excessive alcohol intake, physical and emotional stress, dehydration, and poor anti-seizure drug (ASD) compliance along with sleep deprivation that results in the perfect storm leading to break-through seizure in a patient with epilepsy.

## RELATIONSHIP BETWEEN INTERICTAL EPILEPTIFORM DISCHARGES AND SLEEP STAGES

The frequency of interictal epileptiform discharges (IEDs) also varies according to sleep stages. IEDs are more common during sleep than in the awake state, with some patients showing discharges only during sleep. Their frequency is highest during slow-wave sleep with REM sleep characterized by a paucity of discharges.[18] IEDs also increase after sleep deprivation, and some ASDs may decrease their frequency.[19]

## RELATIONSHIP BETWEEN SEIZURE CONTROL AND SLEEP QUALITY

Sleep and epilepsy make for frequent but incompatible bedfellows. Poor sleep quality, whether the result of poor sleep hygiene, poorly entrained circadian rhythm, or caused by primary sleep disorders such as OSA or restless leg syndrome, results in sleep fragmentation, which lowers seizure threshold and can cause seizures. Poorly controlled epilepsy with frequent nocturnal seizures in turn leads to disruption of sleep architecture, poor sleep quality, cognitive and behavioral impairment, and reduced quality of life. This is a Catch-22 situation further underscoring the importance of recognizing the complex interaction between sleep, sleep disorders, and epilepsy. Improving the sleep quality of patients with epilepsy and treating underlying sleep disorders such as OSA and restless leg syndrome may improve seizure control. Better control of nocturnal seizures in epilepsy patients may improve their sleep and quality of life.

## EFFECTS OF ANTISEIZURE MEDICATIONS ON SLEEP

Antiseizure medications may affect sleep architecture and alter sleep efficiency in positive and negative ways independent of their anticonvulsant effect[20]; this is especially significant for ASDs such as clobazam belonging to the 1,5-benzodiazepine class of drugs and benzodiazepines such as clonazepam and lorazepam. Clobazam causes less sedation than traditional 1,4 benzodiazepine derivatives such as lorazepam and is dosed usually once a day at night due to its sedative effect. Benzodiazepines and barbiturates reduce sleep latency and decrease REM sleep. Lamotrigine, a popular broad-spectrum ASD, on the other hand causes insomnia, and evening dose ideally should be administered a few hours before bedtime. Newer ASDs such as levetiracetam, lacosamide, and brivaracetam seem to be less disruptive to sleep but many have not been systematically studied. Not much is known about the detailed effects of ASDs on sleep architecture, even less is known about the mechanisms by which ASDs cause such effects. Some ASDs such as valproate cause weight gain, which may exacerbate preexisting OSA. Others such as topiramate cause weight loss and may be helpful in an obese OSA patient with coexisting epilepsy. Mood-stabilizing ASDs such as lamotrigine and valproate may be helpful in patients who suffer from psychophysiological insomnia. Chronopharmacology of ASDs has not been systematically studied, and there is limited evidence to suggest that dosing some ASDs based on circadian rhythms may improve absorption and result in better seizure control at lower doses.[21]

## EFFECTS OF SEDATIVE-HYPNOTIC MEDICATIONS ON SEIZURES

Sleep disorders such as insomnia and restless leg syndrome in addition to OSA frequently co-exist in patients with epilepsy. These disorders are treated with sedative-hypnotic medications such as benzodiazepines (clonazepam, lorazepam, diazepam, temazepam), zolpidem, zaleplon, opiates, trazodone, and dopamine agonists that may interact with ASDs; this should be kept in mind when prescribing these medications in a patient with comorbid epilepsy. Benzodiazepines are highly effective as seizure rescue medication when used on demand. Nightly use for insomnia though causes tolerance and dependence, and abrupt discontinuation risks withdrawal seizures.

## RELATIONSHIP BETWEEN SLEEP DISORDERS AND SUDDEN UNEXPECTED DEATH IN A PERSON WITH EPILEPSY

Sudden unexpected death in a person with epilepsy (SUDEP) is defined as the sudden, unexpected, witnessed, or unwitnessed death of a patient with epilepsy with or without evidence of a seizure in which the postmortem examination does not reveal structural, toxicologic, traumatic, or drowning as the cause of death.[22] SUDEP most often occurs in sleep with patients frequently found unresponsive in a prone position in bed. The contribution of comorbid sleep disorders such as central sleep apnea (CSA) and OSA to the risk of SUDEP is indetermined but suspected (**Fig. 1**).[23] Several mechanisms for SUDEP have been postulated. One suspected cause is peri-ictal and postictal apnea trigged by the seizure, leading to decreased ventilation and cardiac arrhythmia. The contribution of co-existing and untreated OSA to this is yet unknown. Patients with OSA exhibit lower heart rate variability and sympathovagal imbalance, which suggests that the disease might play a role in the pathophysiology of at least some SUDEP cases. Likely abnormal breathing patterns triggered by CSA and OSA play a role in the cascade of events that finally culminates in SUDEP.[24]

## RELATIONSHIP BETWEEN OBSTRUCTIVE SLEEP APNEA AND EPILEPSY

Obstructive sleep apnea defined as AHI of 5 or greater shares a complex bidirectional relationship with epilepsy and frequently co-exists. Untreated OSA by causing nocturnal hypoxia, disruption of sleep architecture, sleep fragmentation, and decreased sleep efficiency is postulated to be a trigger for seizures and may contribute to worsening seizure control and in some cases refractory epilepsy. Many studies have associated presence of OSA with increased frequency of nocturnal seizures, refractory epilepsy, and even status epilepticus.[25–28]

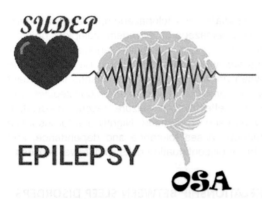

**Fig. 1.** Personal picture; no copyright restrictions. (Modified picture from "https://www.sleepbetterny.com/tag/obstructive-sleep-apnea/".)

One study based on a screening questionnaire demonstrated patients with temporal lobe epilepsy at higher risk for sleep apnea than those with nontemporal lobe epilepsy.[29] Studies have also demonstrated that patients with epilepsy with comorbid OSA have higher rate of IEDs than in the general population.[30] Patients with epilepsy with OSA are more likely to experience seizures during the night as compared with patients with epilepsy without OSA. Rashed and colleagues looked at the association between refractory epilepsy and OSA. Sixty patients with epilepsy, 30 patients with controlled epilepsy, and 30 patients with refractory epilepsy were studied with overnight polysomnogram, sleep EEG, and Sleep Apnea Sleep Disorders Questionnaire. The frequency of OSA was found to be 10% in patients with controlled epilepsy, whereas in patients with refractory epilepsy it was 16.7%.[31] Although this was determined to be statistically insignificant, older patients with early onset of epilepsy and longer duration of epilepsy had higher AHI, suggesting a causal association between refractory epilepsy and OSA. In this study, older age, early onset, and longer duration of epilepsy were determined to be independent risk factors for the OSA in patients with refractory epilepsy. Some studies have suggested that epilepsy may increase the risk of OSA and aggravate it.[32] Patients with epilepsy have been found to have higher frequency and grade of OSA. Whether better control of seizures results in improvement in OSA in these is not known.

Seizures have been implicated as a source of central apneas. In animal models seizure-induced respiratory inhibition and respiratory arrest has been demonstrated. Brainstem serotonergic systems regulate cardiorespiratory changes during the peri-ictal and post-ictal periods.[32] Suppression of these systems lead to impaired cardiorespiratory function in seizures. How seizures precipitate OSA by impairing upper airway control though remains unclear.

Continuous positive airway pressure (CPAP) is the treatment of choice for moderate to severe OSA.[33] Although CPAP has no side effects, a sizable number of patients initially find it uncomfortable, leading to poor compliance. Multiple studies though have consistently shown the benefits of treating OSA with CPAP to improve seizure control irrespective of changes to ASDs.[34,35] The studies though lack control groups, and hence, the influence of confounding factors and placebo effect cannot be excluded. Vendrame and colleagues, in a retrospective study of 41 patients, compared seizure frequency in patients who were compliant with CPAP therapy (n = 28) with that in those who were not (n = 13; <21 days per month and <4 h per day of CPAP use) for at least 6 months. In the CPAP compliant group, seizure frequency decreased on average from 1.8 to 1.0 per month, whereas in the noncompliant group seizure frequency decreased from 2.1 to 1.8. Fifty-seven percent of the compliant group became seizure free compared with 23% of the noncompliant group.[36] In a randomized controlled trial of 68 patients using therapeutic versus sham CPAP, use of CPAP produced improvement in seizure control with seizure freedom in 20%.[35] Hollinger and colleagues retrospectively reviewed the database of their sleep center to identify patients with sleep apnea and epilepsy comorbidity. Characteristics of seizure disorder (epilepsy), sleep history, presence of excessive daytime sleepiness via Epworth Sleepiness Scale (ESS), and polysomnographic data were reviewed. The effect of CPAP on seizure reduction was then prospectively analyzed after a median interval of 26 months (range: 2–116 months) from the diagnosis of OSA. OSA was found in 29 patients with epilepsy (25 men and 4 women) with a median age of 56 years (range: 37–79 years). The median AHI was 33 (range: 10–85), the oxygen desaturation index was 12 (range 0–92), and 52% of the patients had an ESS score greater than 10. The investigators in their cohort found that in 27 patients, epilepsy appeared 1 month to 44 years before the diagnosis of OSA. In 21 patients, the appearance of OSA symptoms coincided with a clear increase in seizure frequency or the first appearance of a status epilepticus event. In 12 patients good compliance with CPAP treatment led to a significant reduction of both ESS scores and seizure frequency in 4 patients.[37] Chihorek and colleagues studied the association of OSA with seizure occurrence in older adults (>50 years of

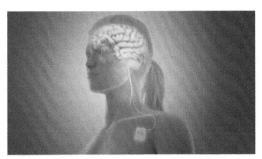

**Fig. 2.** Vagus nerve stimulator. (Vagus nerve stimulation, Scientific Animations. *From*: https://www.scientificanimations.com/wp-content/uploads/2018/02/Vagus-nerve-stimulation.jpg. Licensed under CC BY SA 4.0.)

age) with epilepsy and found that older adults with late-onset or worsening seizures had significantly higher AHI than patients who were seizure free when controlling for other factors such as age, body mass index, neck circumference, number of ASDs currently used, and frequency of nocturnal seizures concluding that OSA is associated with seizure exacerbation in older adults with epilepsy.[38] Other investigators have reported impressive responder rates (>50% seizure reduction) in studies of CPAP for OSA in patients with epilepsy.[35] Studies looking at treatment of OSA in children also reveal marked reduction in seizure frequency.[39]

Studies show CPAP therapy causing reduction in the rates of abnormal IEDs not just during sleep but also during wakefulness.[30] The marked reduction in seizure frequency and IEDs with CPAP therapy support the notion that sleep fragmentation and hypoxia caused by OSA may be contributing to epileptogenicity. The efficacy of other treatments of OSA in patients with epilepsy such as use of mandibular advancement device and surgery such as uvulopalatopharyngoplasty has neither been systematically nor extensively studied. In children, tonsillectomy and adenoidectomy are frequent treatments of OSA. It is unclear whether this surgery results in improved seizure control in pediatric patients with epilepsy although some uncontrolled retrospective studies suggest a beneficial effect.[40]

The VNS (LivaNova, Inc, CO, USA) has been used as an adjunctive treatment of patients with medically refractory epilepsy since 1997 (**Fig. 2**).[41] Some studies have raised concern that VNS therapy may worsen preexisting OSA.[42] The following mechanisms have been postulated. Stimulation of peripheral vagal afferents activates motor efferents with cell bodies in the dorsal motor nucleus of the vagus nerve and in the nucleus ambiguous, thus altering neuromuscular transmission to the upper airway muscles of the pharynx and larynx producing upper airway narrowing and obstruction. Modulation of central projections to the brainstem reticular formation by VNS may alter the rate and depth of respiration. VNS can cause central apneas, obstructive hypopneas, and obstructive apneas. Cases of laryngeal stridor have also been reported, and it is recommended that patients be observed for 15 minutes after stimulation parameter changes.[43,44] Louis and colleagues reported a patient with VNS implantation for medically refractory nonlesional extratemporal partial epilepsy who developed sleep-related stridor after output current was increased to 1.0 mA.[45] During a subsequent overnight polysomnography snoring and stridor stopped completely during VNS deactivation and recurred immediately following VNS reactivation. VNS output current was reduced to 0.5 milliamps, and this completely abolished stridor and snoring. VNS is a semi-closed loop neuromodulator. Once the device is turned on, it sends up current via the left vagus nerve and continues to do so day and night based on the selected parameters namely output current (mA), pulse width, time on, and time off. When it activates during sleep, it may cause reduction in airflow and respiratory effort producing or worsening OSA. VNS also increases REM sleep and may prevent effective CPAP titration.[46] Therefore, it is recommended to have the VNS device turned off to help find effective CPAP pressure during CPAP titration study.[47] Patients with epilepsy should then undergo polysomnography with the VNS turned on, and if OSA persists, either VNS stimulation parameters or CPAP pressure should be adjusted; this requires close coordination between the epileptologist and the sleep specialist. Whether other neuromodulation devices used in patients with refractory epilepsy such as RNS (NeuroPace, Inc, CA, USA) and DBS (Medtronic, Inc, Minneapolis, MN, USA) adversely affect OSA and CPAP titration is not known at this moment.

There are a handful of anecdotal case reports in which resective epilepsy surgery has resulted in resolution or improvement of sleep-disordered breathing.[48] It is unclear whether the improvement is on account of better seizure control or some underlying common mechanism.

Currently there are no consensus guidelines on whether all or some epilepsy patients warrant polysomnography to rule out or rule in OSA. Patients with epilepsy frequently complain of excessive daytime sleepiness and fatigue and American College of Physicians recommends sleep study testing for patients with unexplained sleepiness.[49] If daytime sleepiness (ESS >10) and fatigue in patients with epilepsy cannot be attributed to their seizures or side effects of ASDs, OSA and restless leg syndrome should be considered and ruled out. Polysomnography should also be considered in patients with epilepsy who fail to respond to conventional ASDs and who are obese and have a large neck circumference.

Given the high prevalence of OSA in patients with epilepsy, screening all patients with epilepsy for OSA and treating with nasal CPAP when appropriate is justified.

## SUMMARY

Epilepsy and OSA are intimate but incompatible bedfellows having a complex and bidirectional relationship that affects each other and adversely affects seizure control, OSA severity, and quality of life. Large multicentric studies with randomized placebo-controlled designs and comparing CPAP versus sham CPAP should be carried out to further elucidate the complex interaction of OSA and epilepsy.

## CLINICS CARE POINTS

---

- In every patient with epilepsy, take a focused sleep history.
- When treating patients with epilepsy, especially medically refractory epilepsy, evaluate for coexisting sleep disorder such as obstructive sleep apnea.
- Patients with epilepsy with VNS should have the device turned off to help find effective CPAP pressure during CPAP titration study.

---

## DISCLOSURE

N.K. Sethi serves as Associate Editor, The Eastern Journal of Medicine and Chief Medical Officer to the New York State Athletic Commission (NYSAC).

## REFERENCES

1. Fiest KM, Sauro KM, Wiebe S, et al. Prevalence and incidence of epilepsy: a systematic review and meta-analysis of international studies. Neurology 2017;88:296–303.
2. Krauss G. Epilepsy is not resolved. Epilepsy Curr 2014;14:339–40.
3. International League against Epilepsy definition and classification of epilepsy. Available at: https://www.ilae.org/guidelines/definition-and-classification.
4. Katyayan A, Diaz-Medina G. Epilepsy: epileptic syndromes and treatment. Neurol Clin 2021;39:779–95.
5. Singh G, Sander JW. The global burden of epilepsy report: Implications for low- and middle-income countries. Epilepsy Behav 2020;105:106949.
6. Haerer AF, Anderson DW, Schoenberg BS. Prevalence and clinical features of epilepsy in a biracial United States population. Epilepsia 1986;27:66–75.
7. Rincon N, Barr D, Velez-Ruiz N. Neuromodulation in drug resistant epilepsy. Aging Dis 2021;12:1070–80.
8. Senaratna CV, Perret JL, Lodge CJ, et al. Prevalence of obstructive sleep apnea in the general population: a systematic review. Sleep Med Rev 2017;34:70–81.
9. Rundo JV. Obstructive sleep apnea basics. Cleve Clin J Med 2019;86(9 Suppl 1):2–9.
10. Herman ST, Walczak TS, Bazil CW. Distribution of partial seizures during the sleep–wake cycle: differences by seizure onset site. Neurology 2001;56:1453–9.
11. Ferri R, Rundo F, Silvani A, et al. REM sleep EEG Instability in REM sleep behavior disorder and clonazepam effects. Sleep 2017;40(8).
12. Mirzoev A, Bercovici E, Stewart LS, et al. Circadian profiles of focal epileptic seizures: a need for reappraisal. Seizure 2012;21:412–6.
13. Combi R, Dalprà L, Tenchini ML, et al. Autosomal dominant nocturnal frontal lobe epilepsy–a critical overview. J Neurol 2004;251:923–34.
14. Muzio MR, Cascella M, Al Khalili Y. Landau Kleffner syndrome. In: StatPearls [Internet]. Treasure Island (FL). StatPearls Publishing; 2022.
15. Singhal NS, Sullivan JE. Continuous spike-wave during slow wave sleep and related conditions. ISRN Neurol 2014;2014:619079.
16. Graziosi A, Pellegrino N, Di Stefano V, et al. Misdiagnosis and pitfalls in Panayiotopoulos syndrome. Epilepsy Behav 2019;98(Pt A):124–8.
17. Baykan B, Wolf P. Juvenile myoclonic epilepsy as a spectrum disorder: a focused review. Seizure 2017;49:36–41.
18. Fürbass F, Koren J, Hartmann M, et al. Activation patterns of interictal epileptiform discharges in relation to sleep and seizures: an artificial intelligence driven data analysis. Clin Neurophysiol 2021;132:1584–92.
19. Mohan L, Singh J, Singh Y, et al. Association of interictal epileptiform discharges with sleep and antiepileptic drugs. Ann Neurosci 2016;23:230–4.
20. Shvarts V, Chung S. Epilepsy, antiseizure therapy, and sleep cycle parameters, 2013. Epilepsy Res Treat; 2013:670682.
21. Wang YQ, Zhang MQ, Li R, et al. The Mutual interaction between sleep and epilepsy on the Neurobiological Basis and therapy. Curr Neuropharmacol 2018;16:5–16.

22. Shankar R, Donner EJ, McLean B, et al. Sudden unexpected death in epilepsy (SUDEP): what every neurologist should know. Epileptic Disord 2017;19: 1–9.

23. Sveinsson O, Andersson T, Mattsson P, et al. Clinical risk factors in SUDEP: a nationwide population-based case-control study. Neurology 2020;94: e419–29.

24. Phabphal K, Koonalintip P, Sithinamsuwan P, et al. Obstructive sleep apnea and sudden unexpected death in epilepsy in unselected patients with epilepsy: are they associated? Sleep Breath 2021;25: 1919–24.

25. Somboon T, Grigg-Damberger MM, Foldvary-Schaefer N. Epilepsy and sleep-related breathing Disturbances. Chest 2019;156:172–81.

26. Gogou M, Haidopoulou K, Eboriadou M, et al. Sleep apneas and epilepsy comorbidity in childhood: a systematic review of the literature. Sleep Breath 2015;19:421–32.

27. Jaseja H, Goyal M, Mishra P. Drug-Resistant epilepsy and obstructive sleep apnea: Exploring a Link between the two. World Neurosurg 2021;146: 210–4.

28. Dinkelacker V. Obstructive sleep apnea in drug-resistant epilepsy: a significant comorbidity warranting diagnosis and treatment. Rev Neurol (Paris) 2016;172:361–70.

29. Yildiz FG, Tezer FI, Saygi S. Temporal lobe epilepsy is a predisposing factor for sleep apnea: a questionnaire study in video-EEG monitoring unit. Epilepsy Behav 2015;48:1–3.

30. Pornsriniyom D, Shinlapawittayatorn K, Fong J, et al. Continuous positive airway pressure therapy for obstructive sleep apnea reduces interictal epileptiform discharges in adults with epilepsy. Epilepsy Behav 2014;37:171–4.

31. Rashed HR, Tork MA, El-Nabil LM, et al. Refractory epilepsy and obstructive sleep apnea: is there an association? Egypt J Neurol Psychiatry Neurosurg 2019;55:28.

32. Sahly AN, Shevell M, Sadleir LG, et al. SUDEP risk and autonomic dysfunction in genetic epilepsies. Auton Neurosci 2022;237:102907.

33. Lorenzi-Filho G, Almeida FR, Strollo PJ. Treating OSA: current and emerging therapies beyond CPAP. Respirology 2017;22:1500–7.

34. Pornsriniyom D, Kim Hw, Bena J, et al. Effect of positive airway pressure therapy on seizure control in patients with epilepsy and obstructive sleep apnea. Epilepsy Behav 2014;37:270–5.

35. Malow BA, Foldvary-Schaefer N, Vaughn BV, et al. Treating obstructive sleep apnea in adults with epilepsy: a randomized pilot trial. Neurology 2008;71: 572–7.

36. Vendrame M, Auerbach S, Loddenkemper T, et al. Effect of continuous positive airway pressure treatment on seizure control in patients with obstructive sleep apnea and epilepsy. Epilepsia 2011;52: e168–71.

37. Hollinger P, Khatami R, Gugger M, et al. Epilepsy and obstructive sleep apnea. Eur Neurol 2006;55: 74–9.

38. Chihorek AM, Abou-Khalil B, Malow BA. Obstructive sleep apnea is associated with seizure occurrence in older adults with epilepsy. Neurology 2007;69: 1823–7.

39. Jain SV, Simakajornboon S, Shapiro SM, et al. Obstructive sleep apnea in children with epilepsy: prospective pilot trial. Acta Neurol Scand 2012; 125:e3–6.

40. Saadeh C, Ulualp SO. The effect of tonsillectomy and adenoidectomy on Isolated sleep associated Hypoventilation in children. Laryngoscope 2021; 131:E1380–2.

41. González HFJ, Yengo-Kahn A, Englot DJ. Vagus nerve stimulation for the treatment of epilepsy. Neurosurg Clin N Am 2019;30:219–30.

42. Oh DM, Johnson J, Shah B, et al. Treatment of vagus nerve stimulator-induced sleep-disordered breathing: a case series. Epilepsy Behav Rep 2019;12: 100325.

43. Tami A, Gerges D, Herrington H. Stridor related to vagus nerve stimulator: a case report. Laryngoscope 2021;131:E1733–4.

44. Oliveira Santos M, Bentes C, Teodoro T, et al. Complex sleep-disordered breathing after vagus nerve stimulation: broadening the spectrum of adverse events of special interest. Epileptic Disord 2020; 22:790–6.

45. St Louis EK, Faber K. Reversible sleep-related stridor during vagus nerve stimulation. Epileptic Disord 2010;12:76–80.

46. Upadhyay H, Bhat S, Gupta D, et al. The therapeutic dilemma of vagus nerve stimulator-induced sleep disordered breathing. Ann Thorac Med 2016;11: 151–4.

47. Ebben MR, Sethi NK, Conte M, et al. Vagus nerve stimulation, sleep apnea, and CPAP titration. J Clin Sleep Med 2008;4:471–3.

48. Zanzmera P, Shukla G, Gupta A, et al. Effect of successful epilepsy surgery on subjective and objective sleep parameters–a prospective study. Sleep Med 2013;14:333–8.

49. Qaseem A, Dallas P, Owens DK, et al. Clinical Guidelines Committee of the American College of Physicians. Diagnosis of obstructive sleep apnea in adults: a clinical practice guideline from the American College of Physicians. Ann Intern Med 2014; 161:210–20.

# Cognitive Complaints and Comorbidities in Obstructive Sleep Apnea

Michelle Vardanian, M.Phil[a], Lisa Ravdin, PhD[b],*

## KEYWORDS

- Obstructive sleep apnea • Cognition • Cognitive function • Comorbidities • Neurocognitive function
- Treatment • Cognitive behavioral therapy

## KEY POINTS

- Cognitive complaints are common in patients with obstructive sleep apnea (OSA) and can include reports of decreased attention, executive dysfunction, and memory deficits.
- Although the exact relationship is still unclear, a number of fixed and modifiable risk factors are associated with cognitive dysfunction in OSA.
- OSA increases the risk for a variety of health factors that have been associated with cognitive decline. The morbidity associated with many of these risk factors increases with advanced age.
- PAP therapy has shown some positive impact on cognitive functioning in OSA patients; however, it does not alleviate all cognitive complaints, and some issues persist even with consistent PAP use.
- Complementary and integrative treatment approaches that involve behavioral interventions such as cognitive behavioral therapy or lifestyle changes may serve as practical options to address comorbidities in patients with OSA.

## INTRODUCTION

Obstructive sleep apnea (OSA), the most common breathing-related sleep disorder, manifests as recurring events of airway collapse. OSA-related hypoxia and fragmentary sleep are associated with repeated awakenings, which contribute to nonrestorative sleep and excessive daytime sleepiness.[1] Despite an increasing awareness of this health problem, 80% of individuals remain undiagnosed and untreated.[2]

### Obstructive Sleep Apnea and Associated Morbidities

OSA is associated with increased medical morbidity, notably cardiovascular disease and cerebrovascular events. Hypertension, stroke, diabetes, and kidney disease have all been associated with the presence of OSA[3] and have also been independently linked to cognitive complaints.[4] Gagnon and colleagues[5] found evidence that OSA is a risk factor for mild cognitive impairment and age-related neurocognitive disorders. In a recent review of OSA studies and specific characteristics, Vaessen and colleagues found that a significantly higher number of OSA individuals in the community reported cognitive complaints (eg, vigilance, concentration) as compared to non-OSA individuals.[6] Almost 60% of individuals with OSA were likely to report memory complaints. OSA individuals have are also more likely to report comorbid challenges in other areas of cognition as well, including organization, anxiety, stress, depression, and learning process-related disorders.[1]

[a] Department of Applied Psychology, New York University, 256 Greene Street, 8th Floor, New York, NY 10003, USA; [b] Department of Neurology, Weill Cornell Medicine, 428 East 72nd Street, Suite 500, New York, NY 10021, USA
* Corresponding author.
E-mail address: ldravdin@med.cornell.edu

Sleep Med Clin 17 (2022) 647–656
https://doi.org/10.1016/j.jsmc.2022.07.009

Typical symptoms of individuals who experience OSA include loud snoring, waking up breathless or choking during the night, frequent awakenings throughout the night, and feeling tired even with adequate sleep.[5] Dry throat, headaches, and daytime sleepiness throughout various activities (eg, watching television, driving, and working) are also common in this population and increases with the severity of OSA.[7] There are comorbid complaints that go beyond excessive daytime sleepiness, and some of the most frequent complaints that these individuals report are cognitive in nature and encompass attentional difficulties, short-term memory problems, issues with planning and problem solving, as well as challenges in inhibition, organization, and concentration.[8,9] In addition to cognitive complaints, those with OSA have also reported mood and personality changes, including irritability, increased depressive symptoms, as well as anxiety.[10] There is evidence to suggest OSA may be associated with an earlier age of cognitive decline associated with progression to mild cognitive impairment or Alzheimer disease.[10]

## Mechanisms of Action in Obstructive Sleep Apnea

Mechanisms for the development of cognitive changes in OSA are not well understood and are likely multifactorial given its presence is associated with multiple factors that themselves are associated with cognitive decline. The intermittent hypoxic episodes may affect both brain structure and function that may contribute to cognitive complaints.[11] Evidence suggest that sleep plays an integral role in the production and clearance of brain metabolic products, removing toxic proteins and metabolic waste that amasses during wakefulness, including those that may be involved in dementia pathogenesis.[11] The severity of hypoxia and sleep fragmentation present in OSA is linked to maladaptive and potentially damaging responses (eg, oxidative stress, inflammation, hypertension, dysautonomia, impaired glucose tolerance, and blood–brain barrier dysfunction) that may damage cerebral cells and organelles and make neurons more susceptible to cellular death.[7,11]

The deleterious effects of fragmented sleep on brain health are important to consider for individuals across the life span. For instance, untreated OSA may make the brain more vulnerable to neurodegenerative processes through the gradual changes in brain structure and functioning that occurs[7] via drastic and damaging changes to sleep architecture and intermittent hypoxia.[11] Thus,

OSA may be a risk factor for cognitive decline in neurodegenerative disorders.[1] A recent meta-analysis also indicated that patients diagnosed with Alzheimer disease have a 50% chance of experiencing OSA after their dementia diagnosis.[12] The presence of OSA increases the risk of developing Parkinson disease in women; OSA diagnosed in patients with Parkinson disease has also been observed to increase sleepiness and reduce global cognition.[13]

## Obstructive Sleep Apnea and Cognitive Deficits

### Attention
Several studies have shown that people diagnosed with OSA demonstrate impairments in attentional functioning.[14] Most OSA patients complain of daytime sleepiness that usually occurs when performing tasks that require less attention (ie, reading or watching television, driving). It has been found that individuals with OSA are at an increased risk for vehicle accidents, which has spurred on additional studies related to attentional processes when driving.[15] Studies testing individuals with OSA in driving simulations to measure reaction time and sustained attention have found that OSA individuals consistently performed worse than controls on these instruments.[16] Individuals with OSA have longer reaction times in neuropsychological testing tasks requiring both sustained and selective attention in addition to demonstrating longer reaction times when compared with controls without OSA.[16]

### Executive functioning
A recent meta-analysis reported that 5 domains of executive functioning are impaired in OSA, including inhibition, shifting, working memory, fluid reasoning, and problem-solving.[17] Individuals with OSA make significantly more mistakes or have increased reaction times on cognitive tests that assess this domain when compared with controls without OSA.[18] Individuals with OSA also show an increased number of perseverative responses or needing additional time on tasks that assess shifting, or mental flexibility, when compared with individuals without OSA.[19]

Furthermore, those who are diagnosed with OSA perform poorly on working memory tasks (eg, reciting a string of numbers backwards).[4,5] Indeed, working memory has been found to be one of the most frequently impaired dimensions of executive functioning in people who are diagnosed with OSA,[20,21] although more studies are needed to expand these findings.[5] In studies assessing the performance of people with OSA on tasks that assess problem-solving skills, findings show that these individuals take longer and need more steps to problem-solve effectively.[22]

### Memory

Several lines of evidence suggest that OSA patients have mild but significant memory impairment affecting episodic, procedural, and working memory.[23] Episodic memory is the memorization of verbal or visual information in a spatiotemporal context[5]; this domain of cognitive functioning typically includes immediate recall, total recall over multiple trials or learnings, delayed recall, and recognition memory as relevant assessment tasks. Recent study has found that verbal and visual memory deficits had differing presentations for individuals with OSA, such that verbal memory may be more impaired than visual memory.[24] A recent meta-analysis found that while all memory components were impaired for verbal episodic memory, only immediate and delayed recall components were impaired for visual episodic memory in OSA when compared with controls.[25]

### Depression

Developing research has indicated that mood disorders (eg, depression) may also be linked to the diagnosis of OSA,[18] although the effects of OSA on an individual's emotional functioning remain unclear.[26] Rates of depression are higher in OSA individuals when compared with non-OSA individuals, with more than 60% of patients with OSA experiencing depressive symptoms.[18] Depression is one of the most common mood disorders associated with OSA: those with an OSA diagnosis are 2.4 times more likely to have major depression.[27] The combination of a predisposition to a depressive disorder compounded by OSA may activate latent negative schemas.[28] Regardless of a directional causal relationship between OSA and depression, OSA may exacerbate the damage that depression typically leads to in individuals.[18,26]

### Anxiety and other mood disorders

Research on OSA and other mood disorders is still emerging and needs more work. Preliminary findings have posited that the severity of anxiety symptoms may be dependent on daytime sleepiness rather than nighttime hypoxemia.[26] Yet, more recent literature has found that anxiety may in fact be more common in severe cases of OSA than depression.[29]

Anger is another domain of emotional functioning that needs more research in relation to OSA comorbidities because it may be more strongly linked to hypoxemia.[26]

### Exceptions of Obstructive Sleep Apnea and Cognitive Complaints

An OSA diagnosis does not guarantee cognitive changes, suggesting that synchronous complaints that arise with OSA may be co-occurring impairments or even preexisting issues that have just been noticed with an OSA diagnosis. In clinical practice, the possibility of having OSA and other sleep difficulties are often explored in those presenting cognitive complaints as rule outs for other neurodegenerative or psychological disorders, or as a treatable co-occurring condition that can be the target of intervention. Indeed, some authors have posited that OSA does not actually cause cognitive impairment[30] but rather the comorbidities that commonly present in OSA cases (eg, hypertension, obesity with associated inflammation, diabetes, or metabolic syndrome) are the primary causes of the neurological damage commonly associated with OSA.[9] Clinical experience suggests some comorbid conditions can exacerbate the manifestation of cognitive changes in the context of OSA and vice versa. Identifying and addressing potential contributing factors to cognitive complaints in patients with OSA can lead to improved quality of life and treatment outcomes.

### Factors that Increase Risk of Obstructive Sleep Apnea and Cognitive Comorbidities

There are several fixed and modifiable risk factors associated with the prevalence of OSA that may also increase the risk for cognitive complaints. Understanding the impact of fixed risk factors may help physicians anticipate potential cognitive complaints that could arise based on patients' profiles. Perhaps more importantly, examining modifiable risk factors can sanction health providers to consider and prescribe alternate or additional treatments (in tandem with positive airway pressure [PAP]) that may uniquely address such comorbidities (**Fig. 1** for more details).

### Genetics

Several studies have suggested a strong genetic contribution to sleep disturbances for OSA, hypoxia, and sleep fragmentation.[31] For example, the Apolipoprotein E gene (APOE) has been associated with increased brain vulnerability, suggesting that the presence of this gene may increase the risk of developing OSA as well as cognitive complaints in individuals. A recent study examining the APOE gene in healthy older adults found an association between APOE and poor nighttime sleep quality.[32] APOE has also been identified as a major risk factor for cognitive decline, particularly memory and is most often linked to Alzheimer

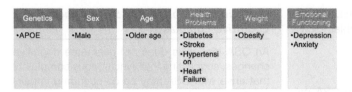

**Fig. 1.** Factors associated with the development of OSA and Comorbid complaints. Note. Columns in blue are fixed factors (ie, not able to be changed voluntarily) while columns in green are modifiable (eg, able to be changed voluntarily).

disease.[33] These mixed results suggest that further research is needed in this area to understand the impact of genes on sleep quality and the development of OSA in tandem with cognitive complaints.

### Sex

One fixed risk factor identified is sex; the available data regarding the prevalence of OSA demonstrate that approximately 11% adult men and 4% adult women hold this diagnosis.[34] The male sex has been found to be a significant predictor of an OSA diagnosis.[35] Although some researchers posit that women may be undiagnosed due to hesitancy in seeking clinical care for these difficulties, there are also physiological differences that increase the chance of OSA in men. Specifically, compared with women, men have a larger, fatter, posterior tongue as well as a longer, collapsible oropharynx (ie, the pharyngeal segment involved in OSA), which both increase the odds of this group developing OSA.[36] Nigro and colleagues found that while men were more significantly likely to report snoring and apnea, and women were more likely to report tiredness and morning headaches, putting them at higher risk of reporting more cognitive complaints.[36] These findings were corroborated in other studies,[35] where women were also more significantly likely to report comorbid depressive symptoms as well as cognitive complaints.

### Age

The dimensions and quality of sleep have increasingly been an area of interest in the health-care field for individuals across the life span and varying ages. OSA is the most prevalent sleep disorder in youth.[37] Children and adolescents with OSA may have reduced sleep quality, resulting in behavioral issues, poor school performance, or daytime sleepiness; studies have also linked OSA in youth to learning and attention deficits as well as behavioral issues.[38] Recent meta-reviews have found that middle-aged adults with OSA experience deficits in multiple cognitive domains, including attention, episodic memory, working memory, and multiple aspects of executive function (eg, task shifting, inhibition, fluid reasoning, and problem-solving), whereas areas of psychomotor abilities,

language, and visuospatial function appear to remain less systematically affected.[8,39] The risk and prevalence of being diagnosed with OSA increases with age.[26] Between the ages of 30 and 49 years, 10% of men and 3% of women are diagnosed, with rates rising to 17% and 9%, respectively, for 50 to 70-year-olds, and increasing to approximately 20% or higher for individuals aged older than 65 years.[9,34] Prevalence rates have been as high as 90% for older adult men.[1]

Age also affects the prevalence rates of OSA and comorbid complaints because aging is associated with changes in both cognition and sleep. Sleep patterns change across the life span, with a steady decline observed in sleep with aging even when medical issues are controlled for.[40] Total sleep time, sleep efficiency, and deep sleep decrease with aging, whereas the number of nocturnal awakenings and time spent awake during the night increase with aging.[41] In fact, sleeping difficulties in old age are highly prevalent and associated with both physical and psychological changes. More than half of all adults aged 55 to 84 years report sleep complaints such as trouble falling asleep or waking up repeatedly at night.[32] A number of cognitive functioning domains also decline with age, including attention, executive cognitive functioning (eg, decision-making, problem-solving, planning and sequencing of responses, multitasking), memory, sensory perception, as well as processing speed.[42]

Older adults have been found to be at risk for acute cognitive complaints or comorbidities when diagnosed with OSA.[5] Additionally, the prevalence of OSA increases in women as they approach menopausal age.[7] Middle-aged adults with severe OSA have been found to be more at risk of cognitive deficits or complaints when compared with younger adults with the same OSA severity.[43,44] However, children with OSA and associated sleep difficulties experience several cognitive and behavioral challenges, including inattention, restlessness, aggressiveness, and learning difficulties.[37]

### Health problems

The relationship between health problems and the development of OSA and cognitive complaints is complex because the direction of effect between these factors remains ambiguous.[33] Specifically, health complications, such as diabetes, hypertension, and cardiovascular disease, put an individual at higher risk of developing OSA as well as developing cognitive deficits.[31,39] However, having OSA as well as cognitive complaints also puts an individual at higher risk for developing health issues, such as hypertension, diabetes, heart failure, stroke, and depression.[45] OSA itself is a risk factor for increased cognitive deficiencies in this population. More severe cases of OSA, which increases the strength of underlying mechanisms (eg, hypoxia, sleep fragmentation, daytime sleepiness) that lead to comorbid cognitive complaints, have also been correlated with an increased likelihood of more severe cognitive complaints and comorbidities.[5] Regardless of the directionality, the risk associated with developing OSA and cognitive complaints through health challenges also increases with age, suggesting that many of these factors are linked and may likely affect one another concurrently.

### Weight
Anatomical abnormalities play a key role in the development of OSA, including obesity, excess regional adipose tissue, enlarged upper airway soft tissues, and craniofacial differences.[46] There is strong evidence that excess weight (eg, morbid obesity) is one of the strongest predictive factors in OSA[47] in both adults as well as children,[48] with obese children recently showing a 46% prevalence of OSA compared with 33% of children seen in a general pediatric clinic.[49] Indeed, obesity may be one of the most important risk factors to monitor for OSA because the majority of OSA patients (ie, approximately two-thirds) are obese and there is an overrepresentation of OSA in obese patients as well.[50] Although the relationship between weight and OSA is still somewhat unclear, specific areas of fat distribution (eg, neck, waist, and abdominal areas with excessive fat tissue) have been specifically related to OSA.[46] Increased body mass index (BMI) in OSA patients has been linked to a decrease in the core abilities of executive functioning, including the reduction of inhibitory control, cognitive flexibility, problem-solving, planning, and perception.[49]

### Emotional functioning
The relationship between mood disorders and OSA is an area that also needs more research because there may be a bidirectional relationship between OSA and emotional functioning and because there are many shared symptoms between these 2 domains.[22] Cognitive complaints,

particularly memory complaints, have often been associated with mood problems in the general population and in nonsleep disorder patients.[6] In these groups, mood problems were shown to be an even stronger predictor for memory complaints than actual impairments in objective memory function. Serotonin levels seem to play an important role in both the development of depression as well as OSA. Gagnon and colleagues found that patients with more severe depressive and anxiety symptoms were more likely to report cognitive complaints.[4] Furthermore, mood problems in patients with OSA were shown to be an even stronger predictor for memory complaints.[6]

## Positive Airway Pressure Therapy and Cognitive Complaints

Treatment of OSA includes PAP, which generally targets OSA by keeping the upper airways open using air pressure, which subsequently decreases hypoxemia and sleep fragmentation.[5] PAP treatment has been observed to provide overall improvement to subjective daytime functioning as well as performance on various cognitive tests that examine neuropsychological functioning after the initiation of treatment[51] (to learn more about PAP therapy and OSA, see other articles published in this volume).

Even though PAP has been shown to improve some physiological and cognitive complaints in individuals who are diagnosed with OSA, comorbid complaints about cognition and mood may not be addressed completely or adequately. Importantly, PAP therapy must be used consistently for at least 6 hours a night for objective symptom reduction, a necessary component that is often not completely adhered to by patients with OSA.[52] As many as 30% of patients refuse this treatment and one-third discontinue its use long-term.[11] In those situations where an individual consistently uses PAP therapy, cognitive complaints may persist. Thus, it is important to explore both the various comorbid cognitive issues that arise in individuals with OSA across the life span as well as how PAP may sufficiently treat these difficulties.

## Effectiveness of Positive Airway Pressure Therapy on Obstructive Sleep Apnea Comorbidities

PAP treatment has been considered the gold standard and first-line treatment of OSA, regardless of what comorbid challenges patients present with. However, research on the effectiveness of PAP treatment on risk factors that increase the prevalence of OSA and comorbid cognitive and mood complaints are complex and limited, with some studies suggesting that PAP may improve or reverse cognitive deficits, whereas others have found no effect.[53] For example, PAP treatment is moderately effective in reducing neurocognitive deficits in patients with excessive daytime sleepiness; however, it has failed in improving impairments in patients who do not experience daytime sleepiness.[54] It is important to consider that alternate interventions may be effective in addressing many of the comorbid cognitive and affective complaints that accompany an OSA diagnosis, especially considering that PAP therapy may not reverse many of the cognitive challenges that accompany an OSA diagnosis.[9] For example, a 12-month randomized trial showed no effect of PAP therapy on cognitive function in adults aged 65 years and older, despite demonstrating improvement in sleepiness.[55]

### Attention

Several studies have shown that PAP therapy can result in significant improvement in attentional issues.[5] However, although there is some recovery in this cognitive domain, PAP has not been able to completely normalize attention processes in individuals diagnosed with OSA.[6] Indeed, both selective and divided attention deficits have been observed even after 3 months of PAP treatment when compared with control groups.[51] Such observations suggest that a portion of attentional complaints witnessed in OSA individuals may be caused by sleep fragmentation and hypoxia; however, treatment of these symptoms may not fully address these cognitive difficulties. It has previously been posited that OSA may cause permanent damage to regions of the brain involved in attention processes[5,51]; however, these claims only consider the effectiveness of PAP treatment in attentional remediation. Importantly, there may be several neuropsychological interventions that, when received in conjunction with PAP therapy, may effectively improve attentional difficulties within this population.

### Executive functioning

Recent reviews have found that PAP treatments lead to a small-to-moderate improvement in executive functions for individuals with OSA and comorbid executive functioning difficulties.[20] For instance, mental flexibility, verbal fluency, and time management are domains that have seen some improvement after PAP therapy.[6] However, areas of behavioral inhibition, working memory, and other areas of executive functioning are not impacted by PAP, even with long-term use of this treatment.[5]

### Memory

There are reports that PAP therapy may be somewhat effective in addressing comorbid memory difficulties in patients with OSA.[5] Indeed, long-term PAP treatment may lead to normal levels of performance in both immediate and delayed memory functioning for both verbal and visual memory domains.[51] However, another recent review found that memory challenges persisted even after PAP treatment.[6]

### Emotional functioning

Some studies argue that independence of depression and OSA is made clear by the fact that depressive symptoms fail to improve following adequate continuous PAP (CPAP) treatment. Other studies argue that depressive symptoms exhibit clinically relevant improvement following CPAP treatment.[4,5] Depressive symptoms are regularly screened in sleep laboratories; however, the typical concern in these situations is the potential misdiagnosis of OSA for depression and the misuse of antidepressant therapy.[18] However, the alternative possibility (ie, OSA being mistakenly diagnosed rather than a mood disorder) is important to consider, especially regarding prescribing the most appropriate and effective treatments for presenting symptoms. For example, mood disorder-related symptoms may lead to worsened executive functioning, which subsequently affects poor job performance, heightening the present mood dysfunction, and leading to poorer sleep quality as well as increased sleep disturbances,[56] which may be even further exacerbated in the presence of OSA, and in turn may lead to a severe decrease in quality of life as well as additional cognitive complaints.[57] When assessing for OSA, physicians should be aware of potentially mistaking a sleep disorder for an underlying depressive or other mood disorder, or in most circumstances, considering the presence of both comorbidly due to their similar phenotypic expressions. Thus, typical treatments for depression may alleviate many of the symptoms that patients with comorbid complaints experience.

### Supplemental Treatments for Comorbid Cognitive Complaints in Obstructive Sleep Apnea

There are several treatment options that may serve as effective complements to PAP therapy that can prevent or intervene cognitive complaints in order to reduce this morbidity in OSA patients (**Fig. 2**). Generally, research studies have demonstrated a close relationship between stress and sleep disturbances in both healthy and clinical populations.[57] Regardless of the specific cause, many

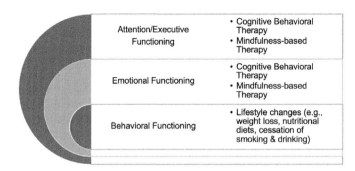

Fig. 2. Suggested supplemental interventions for comorbid complaints in OSA.

| Attention/Executive Functioning | • Cognitive Behavioral Therapy<br>• Mindfulness-based Therapy |
| Emotional Functioning | • Cognitive Behavioral Therapy<br>• Mindfulness-based Therapy |
| Behavioral Functioning | • Lifestyle changes (e.g., weight loss, nutritional diets, cessation of smoking & drinking) |

adults with OSA experiencing cognitive morbidities may benefit from early intervention using psychotherapeutic and neuropsychological treatment approaches.

There is consistent evidence that cognitive behavioral therapeutic approaches have been effective for individuals who experience various cognitive challenges that arise in psychological disorders, including anxiety-related and depression-related disorders across their life span.[58] Cognitive behavioral therapy (CBT), which aims to develop behavioral strategies to compensate for core neuropsychiatric deficits and to change dysfunctional thinking styles,[59] is effective in reducing stress, anxiety, difficulties with attention, executive functioning, as well as sleep hygiene. Researchers have indicated that cognitive complaints can be reduced by CBT that incorporates specific sleep intervention approaches.[60] CBT for insomnia is one such approach because it aims to change dysfunctional thoughts and behavior patterns in individuals through a combination of several components including stimulus control, sleep restriction, cognitive therapy, sleep hygiene, sleep education, and relaxation techniques.[61] It has demonstrated strong effectiveness regarding improving sleep in a variety of settings and populations.[62]

Mindfulness-based cognitive therapy ,[63] acceptance and commitment therapy,[64] and mindfulness meditation training are all psychotherapy approaches that emphasize a compassionate and nonreactive attitude toward one's thoughts, emotions, and body state. These alternative psychotherapeutic approaches have also been shown to be effective in alleviating clinical symptoms of stress, anxiety, and sleep disturbances and may be viable concurrent treatments for physicians to consider prescribing to patients struggling with OSA and comorbid cognitive complaints.[65] Mindfulness interventions have also been adapted for parents of children as well as adolescents with behavioral and cognitive difficulties with a growing body of evidence on its effectiveness for both (eg, observed reductions in externalizing, internalizing, executive functioning, and attention problems).[66]

Behavior parent training (BPT),[67] a widely tested evidence-based treatment of disruptive behavior disorders in youth, may be a viable intervention for families with children who are diagnosed with OSA and experience concurrent cognitive or behavioral challenges.[68] BPT primarily emphasizes social contingencies in which the parent provides positive reinforcement for the child's desirable or prosocial behavior and ignores or provides undesirable consequences for challenging behavior by nonphysical discipline techniques such as the removal of privileges or time out.[67]

Finally, lifestyle changes, including weight and dietary management, may be especially effective in managing comorbid cognitive complaints in patients with OSA and promoting brain health.[69] As previously stated, increased BMI is a risk factor for OSA as well as cognitive complaints. Weight management and healthy nutritional regiments are thus feasible and appropriate interventions in the management of both OSA and cognitive morbidities occurring in these populations.[50] Additionally, other changes in lifestyle, such as decreasing or ceasing smoking, drinking alcohol, and using sedatives, are important recommendations for individuals who have both OSA and cognitive comorbidities because some central nervous system depressant substances or medications (eg, alcohol, opioids, benzodiazepines) may increase the risk of developing OSA.[70] Such behavioral modifications may result in substantial improvements in comorbid health difficulties as well as quality of life experiences.[71] Intensive lifestyle interventions have been effective in the management of OSA as well as neurodegenerative disorders, resulting in a reduction of OSA-related severity as well as cognitive difficulties.[72]

## SUMMARY

There are a number of fixed and modifiable factors that are associated with cognitive consequences in OSA. Cognitive-behavioral therapy, mindfulness-based therapy, behavior-parent trainings, and lifestyle changes are suggested as complementary treatment approaches to enhance the effects of PAP therapy on OSA and cognitive comorbid complaints.

## CLINICS CARE POINTS

- Mechanisms for development of cognitive changes in OSA are not well understood and are likely multifactorial given its presence is associated with multiple factors that themselves are associated with cognitive decline.

- Lower cognitive functioning in areas such as attention, working memory, executive functions is strongly associated with poorer psychosocial functioning, including quality of social relationships, self-care skills, and independent living.

- More research is needed exploring fixed and modifiable at-risk factors for the development of OSA and cognitive comorbidities, especially in relation to mood disorders and their bidirectional nature with OSA.

- Consider age as an important factor for comorbid cognitive changes when evaluating or treating OSA—this clinical presentation could reflect a risk factor for age-related cognitive disorders.

- PAP therapy can be effective treatment of OSA, but can be supplemented by behavioral and lifestyle interventions that can improve outcomes, especially in patients with comorbid cognitive complaints.

- The coronavirus disease pandemic has affected patients on both the macro-level and micro-level: people's lifestyles have significantly changed, which can further contribute to sleep and lifestyle changes as well as emotional dysfunction and alterations in health-related behaviors (eg, decreased physical activity, increased caffeine consumption, overdependence on maladaptive coping strategies such as alcohol consumption). These factors can increase the likelihood of comorbid cognitive complaints in patients with OSA.

- Behavior change is difficult, requires effort and consistent adherence, and may not necessarily be used despite potentially improved health outcomes. Psychoeducation can include managing expectations and encouraging small step increments in behavior change to promote the use of supplementary interventions and utilization of mental health-care services with the hopes of improving comorbid cognitive symptoms in OSA.

## DISCLOSURE

The authors have nothing to disclose.

## REFERENCES

1. Ferini-Strambi L, Lombardi GE, Marelli S, et al. Neurological deficits in obstructive sleep apnea. Curr Treat Options Neurol 2017;19(4):16.
2. Simpson L, Hillman DR, Cooper MN, et al. High prevalence of undiagnosed obstructive sleep apnoea in the general population and methods for screening for representative controls. Sleep Breath 2013;17(3):967–73.
3. Pedrosa RP, Drager LF, Gonzaga CC, et al. Obstructive sleep apnea: the most common secondary cause of hypertension associated with resistant hypertension. Hypertension 2011;58(5):811–7.
4. Gagnon K, Baril AA, Montplaisir J, et al. Disconnection between self-reported and objective cognitive impairment in obstructive sleep apnea. J Clin Sleep Med 2019;15(3):409–15.
5. Gagnon K, Baril AA, Gagnon JF, et al. Cognitive impairment in obstructive sleep apnea. Pathol Biol 2014;62(5):233–40.
6. Vaessen TJ, Overeem S, Sitskoorn MM. Cognitive complaints in obstructive sleep apnea. Sleep Med Rev 2015;19:51–8.
7. Rosenzweig I, Glasser M, Polsek D, et al. Sleep apnoea and the brain: a complex relationship. Lancet Respir Med 2015;3(5):404–14.
8. Bucks RS, Olaithe M, Eastwood P. Neurocognitive function in obstructive sleep apnoea: a meta-review. Respirology 2013;18(1):61–70.
9. Bucks RS, Olaithe M, Rosenzweig I, et al. Reviewing the relationship between OSA and cognition: where do we go from here? Respirology 2017;22(7):1253–61.
10. Osorio RS, Gumb T, Pirraglia E, et al. Sleep-disordered breathing advances cognitive decline in the elderly. Neurology 2015;84(19):1964–71.
11. Gosselin N, Baril AA, Osorio RS, et al. Obstructive sleep apnea and the risk of cognitive decline in older adults. Am J Respir Crit 2019;199(2):142–8.
12. Emamian F, Khazaie H, Tahmasian M, et al. The association between obstructive sleep apnea and Alzheimer's disease: a meta-analysis perspective. Front Aging Neurosci 2016;12(8):78.
13. Mery VP, Gros P, Lafontaine AL, et al. Reduced cognitive function in patients with Parkinson disease and obstructive sleep apnea. Neurology 2017;88(12):1120–8.
14. Ferini-Strambi L, Marelli S, Galbiati A, et al. Effects of continuous positive airway pressure on cognition and neuroimaging data in sleep apnea. Int J Psychophysiol 2013;89(2):203–12.

15. Jordan AS, McSharry DG, Malhotra A. Adult obstructive sleep apnoea. Lancet 2014;383(9918): 736–47.

16. D'Rozario AL, Field CJ, Hoyos CM, et al. Impaired neurobehavioural performance in untreated obstructive sleep apnea patients using a novel standardised test battery. Front Surg 2018;5:35.

17. Davies CR, Harrington JJ. Impact of obstructive sleep apnea on neurocognitive function and impact of continuous positive air pressure. Sleep Med Clin 2016;11(3):287–98.

18. Vanek J, Prasko J, Genzor S, et al. Obstructive sleep apnea, depression and cognitive impairment. Sleep Med 2020;72:50–8.

19. Caporale M, Palmeri R, Corallo F, et al. Cognitive impairment in obstructive sleep apnea syndrome: a descriptive review. Sleep Breath 2021;25:29–40.

20. Olaithe M, Bucks RS, Hillman DR, et al. Cognitive deficits in obstructive sleep apnea: insights from a meta-review and comparison with deficits observed in COPD, insomnia, and sleep deprivation. Sleep Med Rev 2018;38:39–49.

21. Stewart EM, Landry S, Edwards BA, et al. The bidirectional relationship between sleep and health. Wiley Encyclopedia Health Psychol 2021;4(1st edition):165–88.

22. Seda G, Han TS. Effect of obstructive sleep apnea on neurocognitive performance. Sleep Med Clin 2020;15(1):77–85.

23. Joyeux-Faure M, Naegelé B, Pépin JL, et al. Continuous positive airway pressure treatment impact on memory processes in obstructive sleep apnea patients: a randomized sham-controlled trial. Sleep Med 2016;24:44–50.

24. Scullin MK, Bliwise DL. Sleep, cognition, and normal aging: integrating a half century of multidisciplinary research. Perspect Psychol Sci 2015;10(1):97–137.

25. Wallace A, Bucks RS. Memory and obstructive sleep apnea: a meta-analysis. Sleep 2013;36(2):203–20.

26. Vitale GJ, Capp K, Ethridge K, et al. Sleep apnea and the brain: neurocognitive and emotional considerations. J Sleep Disord Manag 2016;2(1):8–12.

27. Wheaton AG, Perry GS, Chapman DP, et al. Sleep disordered breathing and depression among US adults: national health and nutrition examination survey, 2005-2008. Sleep 2012;35(4):461–7.

28. Acker J, Richter K, Piehl A, et al. Obstructive sleep apnea (OSA) and clinical depression—prevalence in a sleep center. Sleep Breath 2017;21(2):311–8.

29. Macey PM, Woo MA, Kumar R, et al. Relationship between obstructive sleep apnea severity and sleep, depression and anxiety symptoms in newly-diagnosed patients. PLoS One 2010;5(4): e10211.

30. Devita M, Montemurro S, Ramponi S, et al. Obstructive sleep apnea and its controversial effects on cognition. J Clin Exp Neuropsychol 2017;39(7):659–69.

31. Varvarigou V, Dahabreh IJ, Malhotra A, et al. A review of genetic association studies of obstructive sleep apnea: field synopsis and meta-analysis. Sleep 2011;34(11):1461–8.

32. Camargos EF, Goncalves ID, Bretones LA, et al. Evidence for a contribution of the APOE (but not the ACE) gene to the sleep profile of non-demented elderly adults. Int J Mol Epidemiol 2019;10(4):59.

33. Gaeta AM, Benítez ID, Jorge C, et al. Prevalence of obstructive sleep apnea in Alzheimer's disease patients. J Neurol 2019;12:1.

34. Peppard PE, Young T, Barnet JH, et al. Increased prevalence of sleep-disordered breathing in adults. Am J Epidemiol 2013;177(9):1006–14.

35. Bostan OC, Akcan B, Saydam CD, et al. Impact of gender on symptoms and comorbidities in obstructive sleep apnea. Eur J Emerg Med 2021;53(1):34.

36. Nigro CA, Dibur E, Borsini E, et al. The influence of gender on symptoms associated with obstructive sleep apnea. Sleep Breath 2018;22(3):683–93.

37. Cardoso CR, Roderjan CN, Cavalcanti AH, et al. Effects of continuous positive airway pressure treatment on aortic stiffness in patients with resistant hypertension and obstructive sleep apnea: a randomized controlled trial. J Sleep Res 2020;29(4): e12990.

38. Gipson K, Lu M, Kinane TB. Sleep-disordered breathing in children. Pediatr Rev 2019;40(1):3.

39. Leng Y, McEvoy CT, Allen IE, et al. Association of sleep-disordered breathing with cognitive function and risk of cognitive impairment: a systematic review and meta-analysis. JAMA Neurol 2017;74(10): 1237–45.

40. Li J, Vitiello MV, Gooneratne NS. Sleep in normal aging. Sleep Med Clin 2018;13(1):1.

41. Gulia KK, Kumar VM. Sleep disorders in the elderly: a growing challenge. Int Psychogeriatr 2018;18(3): 155–65.

42. Murman DL. The impact of age on cognition. In: Seminars in hearing, vol. 36. Thieme (New York): Thieme Medical Publishers; 2015. p. 111–21. No. 03.

43. Yaffe K, Falvey CM, Hoang T. Connections between sleep and cognition in older adults. Lancet Neurol 2014;13(10):1017–28.

44. Cardoso TD, Pompéia S, Miranda MC. Cognitive and behavioral effects of obstructive sleep apnea syndrome in children: a systematic literature review. Sleep Med 2018;46:46–55.

45. Garbarino S, Guglielmi O, Sanna A, et al. Risk of occupational accidents in workers with obstructive sleep apnea: systematic review and meta-analysis. Sleep 2016;39(6):1211–8.

46. Sutherland K, Takaya H, Qian J, et al. Oral appliance treatment response and polysomnographic phenotypes of obstructive sleep apnea. J Clin Sleep Med 2015;11(8):861–8.

47. Joosten SA, Hamilton GS, Naughton MT. Impact of weight loss management in OSA. Chest 2017; 152(1):194–203.

48. Romero-Corral A, Caples SM, Lopez-Jimenez F, et al. Interactions between obesity and obstructive sleep apnea: implications for treatment. Chest 2010;137(3):711–9.

49. Ribeiro OR, do Carmo I, Paiva T, et al. Body mass index and neuropsychological and emotional variables: joint contribution for the screening of sleep apnoea syndrome in obese. Sleep Sci 2021;14(1): 19.

50. Tuomilehto H, Seppä J, Uusitupa M. Obesity and obstructive sleep apnea–clinical significance of weight loss. Sleep Med Rev 2013;17(5):321–9.

51. Lau EY, Eskes GA, Morrison DL, et al. Executive function in patients with obstructive sleep apnea treated with continuous positive airway pressure. J Int Neuropsychol Soc 2010;16(6):1077–88.

52. Saconi B, Polomano RC, Compton PC, et al. The influence of sleep disturbances and sleep disorders on pain outcomes among veterans: a systematic scoping review. Sleep Med Rev 2021;56:101411.

53. Dalmases M, Solé-Padullés C, Torres M, et al. Effect of CPAP on cognition, brain function, and structure among elderly patients with OSA: a randomized pilot study. Chest 2015;148(5):1214–23.

54. Zhou J, Camacho M, Tang X, et al. A review of neurocognitive function and obstructive sleep apnea with or without daytime sleepiness. Sleep Med 2016;23:99–108.

55. McMillan A, Bratton DJ, Faria R, et al. Continuous positive airway pressure in older people with obstructive sleep apnoea syndrome (PREDICT): a 12-month, multicentre, randomised trial. Lancet Respir Med 2014;2(10):804–12.

56. Linton SJ, Kecklund G, Franklin KA, et al. The effect of the work environment on future sleep disturbances: a systematic review. Sleep Med Rev 2015; 23:10–9.

57. Eskildsen A, Fentz HN, Andersen LP, et al. Perceived stress, disturbed sleep, and cognitive impairments in patients with work-related stress complaints: a longitudinal study. Stress 2017;20(4): 371–8.

58. Brenninkmeijer V, Lagerveld SE, Blonk RW, et al. Predicting the effectiveness of work-focused CBT for common mental disorders: the influence of baseline self-efficacy, depression and anxiety. J Occup Rehabil 2019;29(1):31–41.

59. Pettersson R, Söderström S, Edlund-Söderström K, et al. Internet-based cognitive behavioral therapy for adults with ADHD in outpatient psychiatric care: a randomized trial. J Atten Disord 2017;21(6): 508–21.

60. Willert MV, Thulstrup AM, Hertz J, et al. Sleep and cognitive failures improved by a three-month stress management intervention. Int J Stress Manag 2010;17(3):193.

61. Natsky AN, Vakulin A, Chai-Coetzer CL, et al. Economic evaluation of cognitive behavioural therapy for insomnia (CBT-I) for improving health outcomes in adult populations: a systematic review. Sleep Med Rev 2020;54:101351.

62. Koffel EA, Koffel JB, Gehrman PR. A meta-analysis of group cognitive behavioral therapy for insomnia. Sleep Med Rev 2015;19:6–16.

63. Tickell A, Ball S, Bernard P, et al. The effectiveness of mindfulness-based cognitive therapy (MBCT) in real-world healthcare services. Mindfulness 2020; 11(2):279–90.

64. Hayes SC, Strosahl KD, Wilson KG. Acceptance and commitment therapy: the process and practice of mindful change. New York: Guilford Press; 2011.

65. Chiesa A, Calati R, Serretti A. Does mindfulness training improve cognitive abilities? A systematic review of neuropsychological findings. Clin Psychol Rev 2011;31(3):449–64.

66. Van de Weijer-Bergsma E, Formsma AR, de Bruin EI, et al. The effectiveness of mindfulness training on behavioral problems and attentional functioning in adolescents with ADHD. J Child Fam Stud 2012; 21(5):775–87.

67. Chacko A, Jensen SA, Lowry LS, et al. Engagement in behavioral parent training: review of the literature and implications for practice. Clin Child Fam Psychol Rev 2016;19(3):204–15.

68. Vardanian MM, Ramakrishnan A, Peralta S, et al. Clinically significant and reliable change: comparing an evidence-based intervention to usual care. J Child Fam Stud 2020;29(4):921–33.

69. Camolas J. Empowering patients with adequate eating habits in the context of bariatric surgery. Acta Médica Portuguesa 2020;33(6):441.

70. Kolla BP, Foroughi M, Saeidifard F, et al. The impact of alcohol on breathing parameters during sleep: a systematic review and meta-analysis. Sleep Med Rev 2018;42:59–67.

71. Spicuzza L, Caruso D, Di Maria G. Obstructive sleep apnoea syndrome and its management. Ther Adv Chronic Dis 2015;6(5):273–85.

72. Koblinsky, ND, Anderson, ND, Ajwani, F, Parrott, MD, Dawson, D, Marzolini, S, Oh, P, MacIntosh, B, Middleton, L, Ferland, G, Greenwood, CE. Efficacy of the Lifestyle, Exercise and Diet (LEAD) Study: A Cluster Randomized Controlled Trial of a Combined Exercise and Diet Intervention in Older Adults with Vascular Risk Factors and Early Dementia Risk. England: BioMed Central Ltd Pilot and feasibility studies, 2022, Vol.8(1), p.37–37

**UNITED STATES POSTAL SERVICE®**

# Statement of Ownership, Management, and Circulation
### (All Periodicals Publications Except Requester Publications)

| 1. Publication Title | 2. Publication Number | | 3. Filing Date |
|---|---|---|---|
| SLEEP MEDICINE CLINICS | 025 – 053 | | 9/18/2022 |

| 4. Issue Frequency | 5. Number of Issues Published Annually | 6. Annual Subscription Price |
|---|---|---|
| MAR, JUN, SEP, DEC | 4 | $234.00 |

7. Complete Mailing Address of Known Office of Publication (Not printer) (Street, city, county, state, and ZIP+4®)

ELSEVIER INC.
230 Park Avenue, Suite 800
New York, NY 10169

Contact Person
Malathi Samayan

Telephone (Include area code)
91-44-4299-4507

8. Complete Mailing Address of Headquarters or General Business Office of Publisher (Not printer)

ELSEVIER INC.
230 Park Avenue, Suite 800
New York, NY 10169

9. Full Names and Complete Mailing Addresses of Publisher, Editor, and Managing Editor (Do not leave blank)

Publisher (Name and complete mailing address)

DOLORES MELONI, ELSEVIER INC.
1600 JOHN F KENNEDY BLVD. SUITE 1800
PHILADELPHIA, PA 19103-2899

Editor (Name and complete mailing address)

Joanna Collett, ELSEVIER INC.
1600 JOHN F KENNEDY BLVD. SUITE 1800
PHILADELPHIA, PA 19103-2899

Managing Editor (Name and complete mailing address)

Patrick Manley, ELSEVIER INC.
1600 JOHN F KENNEDY BLVD. SUITE 1800
PHILADELPHIA, PA 19103-2899

10. Owner (Do not leave blank. If the publication is owned by a corporation, give the name and address of the corporation immediately followed by the names and addresses of all stockholders owning or holding 1 percent or more of the total amount of stock. If not owned by a corporation, give the names and addresses of the individual owners. If owned by a partnership or other unincorporated firm, give its name and address as well as those of each individual owner. If the publication is published by a nonprofit organization, give its name and address.)

| Full Name | Complete Mailing Address |
|---|---|
| WHOLLY OWNED SUBSIDIARY OF REED/ELSEVIER, US HOLDINGS | 1600 JOHN F KENNEDY BLVD. SUITE 1800 PHILADELPHIA, PA 19103-2899 |

11. Known Bondholders, Mortgagees, and Other Security Holders Owning or Holding 1 Percent or More of Total Amount of Bonds, Mortgages, or Other Securities. If none, check box ► ☐ None

| Full Name | Complete Mailing Address |
|---|---|
| N/A | |

12. Tax Status (For completion by nonprofit organizations authorized to mail at nonprofit rates) (Check one)
The purpose, function, and nonprofit status of this organization and the exempt status for federal income tax purposes:
☒ Has Not Changed During Preceding 12 Months
☐ Has Changed During Preceding 12 Months (Publisher must submit explanation of change with this statement)

PS Form **3526**, July 2014 [Page 1 of 4 (see instructions page 4)] PSN: 7530-01-000-9931 PRIVACY NOTICE: See our privacy policy on www.usps.com.

---

| 13. Publication Title | 14. Issue Date for Circulation Data Below |
|---|---|
| SLEEP MEDICINE CLINICS | JUNE 2022 |

| 15. Extent and Nature of Circulation | | | Average No. Copies Each Issue During Preceding 12 Months | No. Copies of Single Issue Published Nearest to Filing Date |
|---|---|---|---|---|
| a. Total Number of Copies (Net press run) | | | 240 | 192 |
| b. Paid Circulation (By Mail and Outside the Mail) | (1) | Mailed Outside-County Paid Subscriptions Stated on PS Form 3541 (Include paid distribution above nominal rate, advertiser's proof copies, and exchange copies) | 170 | 139 |
| | (2) | Mailed In-County Paid Subscriptions Stated on PS Form 3541 (Include paid distribution above nominal rate, advertiser's proof copies, and exchange copies) | 0 | 0 |
| | (3) | Paid Distribution Outside the Mails Including Sales Through Dealers and Carriers, Street Vendors, Counter Sales, and Other Paid Distribution Outside USPS® | 36 | 29 |
| | (4) | Paid Distribution by Other Classes of Mail Through the USPS (e.g., First-Class Mail®) | 0 | 0 |
| c. Total Paid Distribution (Sum of 15b (1), (2), (3) and (4)) | | | 206 | 168 |
| d. Free or Nominal Rate Distribution (By Mail and Outside the Mail) | (1) | Free or Nominal Rate Outside-County Copies included on PS Form 3541 | 23 | 14 |
| | (2) | Free or Nominal Rate In-County Copies Included on PS Form 3541 | 0 | 0 |
| | (3) | Free or Nominal Rate Copies Mailed at Other Classes Through the USPS (e.g., First-Class Mail) | 0 | 0 |
| | (4) | Free or Nominal Rate Distribution Outside the Mail (Carriers or other means) | 0 | 0 |
| e. Total Free or Nominal Rate Distribution (Sum of 15d (1), (2), (3) and (4)) | | | 23 | 14 |
| f. Total Distribution (Sum of 15c and 15e) | | | 229 | 182 |
| g. Copies not Distributed (See Instructions to Publishers #4 (page #3)) | | | 11 | 10 |
| h. Total (Sum of 15f and g) | | | 240 | 192 |
| i. Percent Paid (15c divided by 15f times 100) | | | 89.95% | 92.30% |

* If you are claiming electronic copies, go to line 16 on page 3. If you are not claiming electronic copies, skip to line 17 on page 3.

PS Form **3526**, July 2014 (Page 2 of 4)

| 16. Electronic Copy Circulation | Average No. Copies Each Issue During Preceding 12 Months | No. Copies of Single Issue Published Nearest to Filing Date |
|---|---|---|
| a. Paid Electronic Copies ► | | |
| b. Total Paid Print Copies (Line 15c) + Paid Electronic Copies (Line 16a) ► | | |
| c. Total Print Distribution (Line 15f) + Paid Electronic Copies (Line 16a) ► | | |
| d. Percent Paid (Both Print & Electronic Copies) (16b divided by 16c × 100) ► | | |

☒ I certify that 50% of all my distributed copies (electronic and print) are paid above a nominal price.

17. Publication of Statement of Ownership

☒ If the publication is a general publication, publication of this statement is required. Will be printed in the DECEMBER 2022 issue of this publication. ☐ Publication not required.

| 18. Signature and Title of Editor, Publisher, Business Manager, or Owner | Date |
|---|---|
| Malathi Samayan - Distribution Controller *Malathi Samayan* | 9/18/2022 |

I certify that all information furnished on this form is true and complete. I understand that anyone who furnishes false or misleading information on this form or who omits material or information requested on the form may be subject to criminal sanctions (including fines and imprisonment) and/or civil sanctions (including civil penalties).

PS Form **3526**, July 2014 (Page 3 of 4) PRIVACY NOTICE: See our privacy policy on www.usps.com.

Printed and bound by CPI Group (UK) Ltd, Croydon, CR0 4YY

03/10/2024

01040365-0008